KETO FOR WOMEN OVER 50

THE ESSENTIAL GUIDE

Table of contents

INTRODUCTION TO KETOGENIC DIET

The Ketogenic Diet is a high-fat eating routine which seems to profit a few people with epilepsy, particularly youngsters. It's anything but an enchantment fix yet one option in contrast to the different anti-epileptic drugs at present accessible. The ketogenic diet offers the benefit of improved seizure control for certain youngsters, and now and again, improved mental sharpness with less meds. The ketogenic diet is frequently viewed as a troublesome routine to follow, be that as it may, with training, and an understanding what the eating routine plans to accomplish, it tends to be reduced to a sensible routine. The fundamental point is to switch the body's essential fuel source from carbohydrates (like bread and sugar) to fats. This is finished by expanding the admission of fats and incredibly decreasing the admission of carbohydrates. The genuine trouble is that the eating regimen is prohibitive to such an extent, that all foods eaten must be weighed out to a tenth of a gram during meal readiness, and a member may not eat anything which isn't "endorsed" by the dietician. The degree of carbohydrates permitted is low so that even the limited quantity of sugar in generally fluid or chewable meds will keep the eating regimen from working. As examples, a run of the mill meal may incorporate some sort of meat with green vegetables cooked with a mayonnaise sauce or a ton of margarine. Overwhelming cream might be remembered for the side for drinking. Another meal may comprise of bacon and eggs with a ton of spread or oil included, and overwhelming cream to drink. A high proportion of fats to carbohydrates must be kept up with a low complete calorie consumption for the eating regimen to be effective.

Fats have been the subject of a great deal of terrible press as of late. What's more many "healthy" foods are promoted with a low fat content...after all "cholesterol slaughters" isn't that right? The fact of the matter is significantly increasingly unpredictable. The facts demonstrate that an excess of fat can prompt arteriosclerosis (blockages of the veins), which can prompt cardiovascular failures or strokes. However, fats additionally have a significant task to carry out in wholesome health. Indeed, even cholesterol in controlled sums is vital and not as terrible as individuals have been instructed.

SHORT HISTORY OF KETOGENIC

The ketogenic diet is anything but another treatment. It has been perceived that if an individual with epilepsy quits eating (fats) their seizures, for the most part, stop. The primary logical research on fasting for the treatment of epilepsy was done in France in 1910. This research revealed that seizures quit during outright fasting. Afterwards, different specialists likewise watched discontinuance of seizures and improvement in mental action during starvation, be that as it may, an individual can't quick inconclusively. In this manner, in 1921 Dr More stunning, at the Mayo Clinic, had a go at utilizing a ketogenic diet to treat patients with epilepsy. He had been utilizing this equivalent eating regimen to draw out ketosis in diabetic patients. At about a similar time Drs Howland and Gamble at the Johns Hopkins Department of Pediatrics saw that "petition and a water diet which likewise included starvation for three to about a month" reduced seizures in a nephew of an educator of pediatrics. Different agents like Dr's Lennox and Cobb at Harvard University likewise started to examine the ketogenic diet.

By 1924, Dr Peterman, at the Mayo Clinic, was utilizing the eating routine normally, and the treatment turned out to be broadly utilized during the 1930s. After World War II, Dr Livingston at Johns Hopkins contemplated just about 1000 patients utilizing the ketogenic diet and announced amazing seizure control. Be that as it may, as more up to date and progressively successful anti-seizure drugs were presented, enthusiasm for the ketogenic diet declined. Around the finish of the 1980s, enthusiasm for the eating routine was resuscitated by Dr John Freeman at Johns Hopkins, who revealed an research in 1992 indicating that the eating routine created total seizure control in 30% of kids with beforehand uncontrolled seizures. One of the kids treated effectively by the Johns Hopkins group was Charlie Abrahams. In appreciation, his folks have made the Charlie Foundation, which has given across the board exposure to the eating regimen, to some degree by making accessible a free videotape.

WHAT IS THE KETOSIS

Ketosis is a procedure that happens when human body needs more carbs to consume for vitality. Rather, it consumes fat and makes substances called ketones, which it can use for fuel.

Ketosis is a metabolic state wherein your body utilizes fat and ketones as opposed to glucose (sugar) as its principal fuel source.

Glucose is put away in your liver and discharged varying for vitality. In any case, after carb consumption has been amazingly low for one to two days, these glucose stores become exhausted. Your liver can make some glucose from amino acids in the protein you eat by means of a procedure known as gluconeogenesis, yet not about enough to address the issues of your cerebrum, which requires a consistent fuel supply.

In ketosis, your body produces ketones at a quickened rate. Ketones, or ketone bodies, are made by your liver from fat that you eat and your own body fat. The three ketone bodies are beta-hydroxybutyrate (BHB), acetoacetate, and CH3)2CO (in spite of the fact that CH3)2CO is, in fact, a breakdown result of acetoacetate).

Your liver really delivers ketones all the time in any event, when eating a higher-carb diet. This happens principally overnight while you rest yet normally just in small sums. Be that as it may, when glucose and insulin levels decline on a carb-limited eating regimen, the liver increases its generation of ketones so as to give vitality to your mind.

When the degree of ketones in your blood arrives at a specific edge, you are viewed as in dietary ketosis. As per driving ketogenic diet analysts Dr Steve Phinney and Dr Jeff Volek, the edge for healthful ketosis is at least 0.5 mmol/L of BHB (the ketone body estimated in the blood).

Albeit both fasting and a keto diet will permit you to accomplish ketosis, just a keto diet is supportable over significant stretches of time. Truth be told, it gives off an impression of being a healthy method to eat that individuals can conceivably follow inconclusively.

BENEFITS OF KETOSIS.

Seeing how our body capacities as far as biochemical procedures will help us is making health evolving steps. For example, admission of a lot of carbohydrates and cholesterol may prompt stroke or coronary episode. Be that as it may, avoiding sugar diet s regularly brings about a response that causes a condition known as ketosis, where the body utilizes put away fat as vitality.

1. Reduces cholesterol levels in the body

Consuming less calories on low sugar foods (carb) reduces elevated cholesterol levels. Eating starch-based weight control plans and less sugar brings down the generation of glucose. Lower cholesterol and carbohydrates levels help hinder age-related maladies.

2. Improves mental keenness

On the off chance that you want to shed somewhere in the range of hardly any pounds without eating fewer carbs, improve your inventiveness, or even take care of basic health problems like indigestion or skin flaws, homeostatic sustenance (otherwise called ketogenic nourishment) may be perfect for you.
3. Helps in weight loss

A substance known as ketone is created when fats are separated to discharge vitality. At first, the ketones framed during this procedure are discharged by the body as pee. In any case, ketones regularly amass in the body prompting a condition known as ketosis. The basic reactions related to this condition incorporate loss of hunger, accordingly is advantageous to individuals trying to shed a couple of pounds.

4. Reduce hunger desires

Ketosis happens when your body is denied of carbohydrates. It utilizes put away fat as vitality and consequently is advantageous on the off chance that you are consuming less calories. Low carb sustenance joined with customary protein admission help to keep your muscles fit. Likewise, low carb nourishment enormously reduces the pace of digestion in your body, which thus reduces hunger desires.

In spite of the fact that there are no disadvantages related to ketosis with respect to weight loss, normal symptoms may incorporate steady fatigue and general tiredness. Also, it can cause liver harm and muscle degeneration.

Forestalling Heart Disease (lower circulatory strain, lower triglycerides, better cholesterol profiles)

Once more, identified with the downstream impacts of keeping blood glucose low and stable, ketogenic abstaining from excessive food intake assists hold with blooding pressure within proper limits and brings down triglyceride levels.

While it might appear to be irrational that eating a higher level of fat in your eating regimen brings down triglycerides, for reasons unknown, the utilization of abundance carbs (particularly fructose) is the key driver of expanding triglycerides.

What's more, with respect to HDL and LDL particles (which the body uses to move fat and cholesterol around), ketogenic eating fewer carbs helps raise HDL ("great cholesterol") and improve the profile of LDL ("terrible cholesterol").

Low-Carb Diets Can Reduce Appetite.

The craving will, in general, is the most exceedingly terrible symptom of consuming less calories.

It is one of the principal reasons why numerous individuals feel hopeless and in the end, surrender.

Be that as it may, low-carb eating prompts a programmed decrease in hunger.

Cutting carbs can naturally reduce your hunger and calorie consumption.

The Low-Carb Diets Can Lead to More Weight Loss at First

Cutting carbs is one of the least difficult and best approaches to shed pounds.

Individuals on low-carb slims down lose more weight, quicker than those on low-fat eating regimens — in any event, when the last are effectively limiting calories.

This is on the grounds that low-carb counts calories act to free overabundance water from your body, bringing insulin levels and driving down to quick weight loss in the primary week or two.

Nearly no matter what, low-carb counts calories lead to more transient weight loss than low-fat eating regimens. In any case, low-carb slims down appear to lose their preferred position in the long haul.

A Large Proportion of Fat Loss Comes From Your Abdominal Cavity

Not all the fat in your body is the equivalent.

Where fat is put away decides how it influences your health and danger of malady.

The two principal types are subcutaneous fat, which is under your skin, and instinctive fat, which collects in your stomach depression and is commonplace for most overweight men.

Instinctive fat will remain in general hotel around your organs. Abundance instinctive fat is related to irritation and insulin opposition — and may drive the metabolic brokenness so basic in the West today.

Low-carb counts calories are extremely viable at decreasing this hurtful stomach fat. A more prominent extent of the fat individuals lose on low-carb eat less carbs appears to originate from the stomach pit.

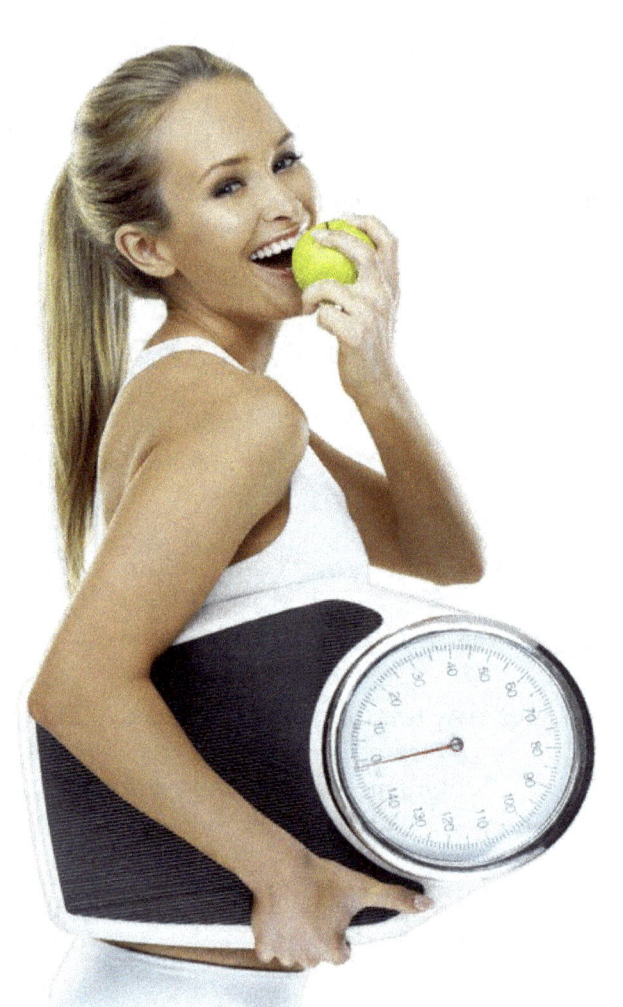

WHY THE KETOGENIC DIET FOR WOMEN OVER 50

Women who experience experienced menopause know the difficulties it brings: crabbiness, expanded fatigue, and weight gain. Fortunately, the keto diet has substantiated itself as a powerful method to shed pounds and improve overall health. Not certain how to start? Continue perusing to discover how to follow keto for women over 50.

Keto for women over 50 assists with diminishing a portion of the reactions of menopause. A portion of the manners in which it helps is: keeping up a healthy weight, decreasing body fat, and improving insight. Here are a couple of subjective benefits:

Equalization Hormones: Most of the indications of menopause experienced by women are because of uneven hormonal characters. The keto diet for women works by normalizing these awkward nature of hormones, for example, estrogen. This empowers you to encounter lesser post-menopausal side effects like hot flashes. Regardless of whether they happen, they are shorter in term and increasingly tolerable. The ketogenic diet additionally balances insulin and directs insulin affectability. This hormone adjusting impact of the keto diet has likewise been demonstrated to treat PMS side effects in more youthful females.

Improve Brain Functions: The hormone estrogen guarantees a smooth inflow of glucose into your mind. Nonetheless, after menopause, the elevated levels of estrogen, in the long run, start to drop thus does the measure of glucose arriving at your mind. On the off chance that you are not getting enough glucose, your mental capacities will begin to decrease. By the accompanying keto diet, the issue of glucose admission is skirted. This prompts upgraded perception and cerebrum capacities.

Increment Sex Drive: The ketogenic diet expands the assimilation of fat-dissolvable nutrients, particularly nutrient D. Being a forerunner of sex hormones, nutrient D guarantees adjusted degrees of testosterone and other sex hormones that could get lopsided because of testosterone.

Improve Sleep: Even a limited quantity of glucose can upset your glucose levels. This prompts low quality of rest. Joined with other menopausal indications, your rest can truly get disturbed as you age. The ketogenic diet adjusts blood glucose levels, and different hormones like cortisol, melatonin, and serotonin guaranteeing an improved rest.

Reduces aggravation: Menopause can build the degree of irritation which can prompt undesirable and difficult side effects. Women over 50 after a keto diet utilizes healthy anti-incendiary fats to reduce irritation and lower torment in your joints and spine.

A KETOGENIC DIET FOR WOMEN OVER 50 YEARS AND HORMONAL RESPONSE

Menopause and weight gain frequently go together gratitude to a mix of hormonal disharmony, more slow digestion and way of life factors.

To accomplish hormone concordance, it takes more than essentially concentrating on one hormone. Along these lines, for the following a month, I will acquaint you with the 4 hormones that could be sabotaging your weight loss endeavours.

Estrogen

Estrogen is certifiably not a solitary hormone; however, a class of hormones. There are three significant Estrogens that women produce – estriol, estradiol and osteon.

Estrogen is one of the significant female sex hormones. Men likewise produce it, yet in littler sums. Truth be told, falling degrees of estrogen add to men's growing waistlines similarly as they do in women, in later years.

Normally higher in women, Estrogen is answerable for forming a lady's remarkable figure. With age, be that as it may, the Estrogen levels decline, prompting women taking on a progressively manly figure.

Estrogen is additionally the hormone that could be raising you the most ruckus in the fat division. At the point when Estrogen levels are out of equalization, they can transform you into a fat creating machine, once in a while at a quick pace, that leaves numerous women sad and baffled.

Estrogen works pair with progesterone. Progesterone has a place with a gathering of steroid hormones called progestogens. Progesterone levels likewise decline in your later years. Low degrees of progesterone can cause side effects, for example, bosom expanding and delicacy, disposition swings, crabbiness, inconvenience resting and water maintenance.

Estrogen and Weight Gain

Estrogen's answerable for expanding fat stockpiling at the hips and thighs, giving the hour-glass shape. Progesterone, when working as one with Estrogen, typically stops the capacity of fat around the abdomen, yet factors can become possibly the most important factor that meddles with this agreeable organization.

Stress can negatively affect progesterone's activity. It prompts weight gain around the gut that is extremely hard to move because of your progesterone levels being fundamentally lower than your Estrogen levels.

Elevated levels of pressure have been appeared to affect progesterone contrarily. Consequently, on the off chance that you discover fat gathering around your midriff, you might need to work at lessening any worry in your life and help hold progesterone levels in line.

Since Estrogen levels decrease in a lady's later years, which prompts the negative impacts related with menopause –, for example, hot flushes and night sweats – a significant number of my customers feel that, without a doubt, having an abundance of Estrogen is something to be thankful for.

At the point when you are Estrogen predominant, the constructive outcomes that progesterone has on the body are blocked. This happens on the grounds that Estrogen overstimulates both the cerebrum and the body.

Impacts, for example, serenity and facilitating liquid maintenance are the two significant, superb benefits of progesterone that are tragically missed by any Estrogen prevailing, nervous, enlarged, focused on lady.

Disarray emerges when you are low in Estrogen however are still Estrogen predominant. Estrogen strength happens when your proportion of Estrogen to progesterone is higher than typical. You need progesterone to hold Estrogen's flighty courses under control.

Numerous progressions during the years paving the way to menopause (perimenopause) are expedited by changing degrees of hormones delivered by the ovaries, essentially estrogen.

Estrogen. As the essential "female" hormone, estrogen advances the development and health of the female conceptive organs and keeps the vagina saturated, versatile (stretchy), and all-around provided with blood. Estrogen levels for the most part, decay during perimenopause, yet they do as such in an unpredictable design. Some of the time, there can be more estrogen present during perimenopause than previously.

Estrogen levels for the most part, decay during perimenopause, yet they do as such in an unpredictable style.

As point by point in the table beneath, the reduced creation of estrogen starting in perimenopause can influence your sexual capacity legitimately, for example, through vaginal dryness. It can likewise do so by implication, like hot flashes and night sweats, which can deplete your vitality and undermine your longing for sex, therefore. These impacts are examined in detail in the

"Reasons for Sexual Problems" segment of this program.

Progesterone and testosterone. Notwithstanding estrogen, levels of different hormones created by the ovaries—progesterone (another female hormone) and testosterone (a male androgen hormone delivered at lower levels in women) are additionally changing during your midlife years, as clarified in the table underneath.

Irregular reductions in progesterone influence menstrual periods more than they influence sexual capacity, yet age-related decreases in testosterone may hose charisma (sex drive) in midlife women, in spite of the fact that this remaining parts controversial. The way that estrogen decays more than testosterone persuades that charisma ought not to decrease at menopause. The decrease in testosterone in women is exclusively age-related, not menopause-related, and starts a long time before perimenopause.

KETOGENIC DIET AS AN ANTI AGING MEASURE FOR WOMEN OVER 50

Here are seven genuine anti-ageing tricks that each lady over 50 should utilize.

Wear a Genuine Smile

Nothing will make you look more established and more worn out than wearing a ceaseless glower. The inverse is likewise valid. A certified grin enacts the entirety of the great muscles in your face and tells the world that you are a certain, cheerful individual.

Grinning can likewise make you more joyful, through a procedure that therapists call the "facial input impact." This is incredible news, in light of the fact that the more joyful you are, the more probable you will be to participate in exercises that keep your body and brain fit as a fiddle.

Invest Energy with Young People

Nothing will cause you to feel 10 years more youthful snappier than playing in the recreation centre with a frozen yoghurt fuelled 5-year old. As I composed already, small children can likewise show us an astonishing sum about taking full advantage of life after 50.

In the event that you don't have small children in your family, why not chip in at nearby youth community or turning into a tutor? Giving back has been appeared to make you more joyful, and it might simply keep you feeling more youthful as well!

Consume Fat the Old Fashion Way

Alright, I get it. Remaining fit as a fiddle truly is more earnestly after 50. It requires duty and order. In any case, on the off chance that we are straightforward with ourselves, we as a whole realize that exercise joined with a healthy eating routine, is the absolute most ideal approach to look and feel energetic.

Here's a simple method to get fit as a fiddle in only one moment daily. Suppose that you need to begin running. Attempt the accompanying.

On a primary day, take a one-minute walk. The following day, stroll for two minutes. Proceed with this procedure until you are strolling for 30 minutes toward the month's end. Presently, begin running for the main moment and strolling for the staying 29. On the off chance that you proceed with this procedure before the second's over a month, you will be running 30 minutes every day. To simple? That is a general-purpose!

Grasp Your Passions

The greater part of our grown-up lives is spent taking care of others. As guardians, we regularly put our kids' needs in front of our own. As representatives, we bolster our associates and chiefs. Presently, in our 50s, it's an ideal opportunity to begin grasping our own interests.

Anti-ageing creams regularly guarantee to give you a "healthy gleam." Well, I guarantee that nothing will make you sparkle more splendid than realizing that you are improving the world a spot, in your own exceptional way.

Quit Helping the Clock

At the point when specialists are working with a patient, they generally attempt to "first do no damage." The equivalent applies to anti-ageing. There are not many, assuming any, ensured anti-ageing medications. In any case, there are a lot of things that will remove a very long time from your life, while making you look more established.

When we arrive at our 50s, it's anything but difficult to expect that "the harm has been finished." Nothing could be further from reality. Indeed, we as a whole, know our concern zones. In the event that you despite everything smoke in your 50s, presently is the ideal time to stop. Peruse progressively about the 4 negative behaviour patterns we should kick in our 50s.

Give Your Skin What it Really Needs.

Your skin is astounding and, generally, it is superbly fit for dealing with itself. Of course, utilizing a characteristic cream will assist with securing dampness in your skin. Be that as it may, generally, all your skin needs to remain healthy is sunscreen, water and a fair eating regimen. In spite of what the enhancement organizations may need you to accept, the ideal approach to get the nutrients your skin needs is to eat a decent eating regimen, with a lot of foods grown from the ground.

Discover Friends Who Make You Laugh

Great companions are a fundamental piece of your "anti-ageing unit" for two reasons. To start with, chuckling is a characteristic state of mind and vitality supporter. With the correct companions on your side, you will be bound to take part in the healthy practices that will keep you feeling healthy.

Second, and all the more significantly, encircle yourself with great companions will remind you to be consistent with yourself. This implies figuring out how to cherish your ageing body. No anti-ageing pill or mixture is going to make you more flawless than you as of now are.

What other "anti-ageing" tips would you offer to women in their 50s? It would be ideal if you join the discussion and "like" and offer this article to prop the discussion up.

TIPS TO LOOSE WEIGHT ON KETO FOR WOMEN OVER 50

For some, individuals, keeping up a healthy weight or losing overabundance body fat can get more diligently as the years pass by.

Unhealthy propensities, a generally stationary way of life, poor dietary decisions, and metabolic changes would all be able to add to weight increase after the age of 50.

Be that as it may, with a couple of straightforward alterations, you can get more fit at any age paying little heed to your physical capacities or restorative analyses.

Here are the 20 most ideal approaches to shed pounds after 50.

1. Figure out how to appreciate quality preparing

In spite of the fact that cardio gets a ton of consideration with regards to weight loss, quality preparing is additionally significant, particularly for more seasoned grown-ups.

As you age, your bulk decreases in a procedure called sarcopenia. This loss of bulk starts around the age of 50 and can slow your digestion, which may prompt weight gain.

After the age of 50, your bulk diminishes by around 1–2% every year, while your muscle quality decreases at a pace of 1.5–5% every year.

In this manner, adding muscle-building exercises to your routine is basic for decreasing age-related muscle loss and advancing a healthy body weight.

Quality preparing, for example, bodyweight exercises and weightlifting, can altogether improve muscle quality and increment muscle size and capacity.

Besides, quality preparing can assist you with getting more fit by diminishing body fat and boosting your digestion, which can build what number of calories you consume for the duration of the day.

2. Group up

Presenting a healthy eating example or exercise routine all alone can be testing. Matching up with a companion, colleague, or relative may give you a superior possibility at adhering to your arrangement and accomplishing your wellbeing objectives.

Individuals who regularly go-to weight loss programs with companions are fundamentally bound to keep up their weight loss over time

Also, working out with companions can reinforce your duty to a work out regime and make practising increasingly pleasant.

3. Sit less and move more

Burning a greater number of calories than you take in is basic to losing abundance body fat. That is the reason being increasingly dynamic for the duration of the day is significant when attempting to get fit.

For instance, sitting at your particular employment for significant stretches of time may block your weight loss endeavours. To balance this, you can turn out to be increasingly dynamic at work by essentially finding a good pace work area and going for a five-minute stroll each hour.

Following your means, utilizing a pedometer or Fit piece can support weight loss by expanding your activity levels and calorie use.

When utilizing a pedometer or Fit piece, start with a practical advance objective dependent on your present movement levels. At that point continuously stir your way up to 7,000–10,000 stages for each day or more, contingent upon your overall health.

4. Knock up your protein consumption

Getting enough top-notch protein in your eating regimen isn't significant for weight loss yet additionally basic for halting or turning around age-related muscle loss.

What number of calories you consume very still, or your resting metabolic rate (RMR), diminishes by 1–2% every decade after you turn 20. This is related to age-related muscle loss.

Be that as it may, eating a protein-rich eating routine can help forestall or even switch muscle loss. Various investigations have additionally indicated that expanding dietary protein can assist you with getting thinner and keep it off in the long haul.

More seasoned grown-ups have higher protein needs than more youthful grown-ups, making it even more essential to include protein-rich foods to your meals and bites.

5. Converse with a dietitian

Finding an eating design that both advances weight loss and feeds your body can be troublesome.

Counselling an enlisted dietitian can assist you with deciding the ideal approach to lose abundance body fat without following an overly prohibitive eating routine. Moreover, a dietitian can support and guide you all through your weight loss venture.

Working with a dietitian to get in shape can prompt essentially preferred outcomes over-grinding away alone, and it might assist you with keeping up the weight loss over time.

6. Cook more at home

Various researches have shown that individuals who get ready and eat more meals at home will, in general, follow a healthier eating routine and weigh not exactly the individuals who don't.

Preparing meals at home permits you to control what goes in — and what remains out — of your recipes. It additionally lets you explore different avenues regarding remarkable, healthy fixings that arouse your curiosity.

On the off chance that you eat most meals out of the house, start by preparing a couple of meals for each week at home, and afterwards step by step increment this number until you're cooking at home more than you eat out.

7. Eat more produce

Vegetables and natural products are stuffed with supplements that are crucial to your health, and including them into your eating routine is a basic, proof-based approach to drop overabundance weight.

For instance, a survey of 10 investigations found that each every day serving increment of vegetables was related with a 0.14-inch (0.36-cm) midsection circuit decrease in women.

Eating foods grown from the ground with lower body weight, reduced abdomen outline, and less body fat.

8. Contract a fitness coach

Working with a fitness coach can particularly profit the individuals who are new to turning out by showing you the right method to exercise to advance weight loss and avoiding damage.

In addition, fitness coaches can persuade you to turn out additional by keeping you responsible. They may even improve your disposition about working out.

9. Depend less on comfort foods

Normally eating accommodation foods, for example, inexpensive food, sweet, and prepared tidbits, is related to the weight put on and may obstruct your weight loss endeavours.

Accommodation foods are regularly high in calories and will, in general, below in significant supplements like protein, fibre, nutrients, and minerals. That is the reason inexpensive food and other handled foods are normally alluded to as "unfilled calories."

Reducing comfort foods and supplanting them with nutritious meals and bites that rotate around supplement entire thick foods is a shrewd method to get in shape.

10. Discover a movement that you love

Finding an exercise routine that you can keep up long haul can be troublesome. This is the reason it's essential to take part in exercises that you appreciate.

For instance, on the off chance that you like gathering exercises, pursue a team activity like soccer or a running club so you can exercise with others all the time.

On the off chance that independent exercises are more your style, have a go at biking, strolling, climbing, or swimming without anyone else.

11. Get checked by a healthcare supplier

On the off chance that you are attempting to get more fit despite the fact that you're dynamic and follow a healthy eating routine, deciding out conditions that may make it hard to shed pounds — like hypothyroidism and polycystic ovarian disorder (PCOS) — might be justified.

This might be particularly valid in the event that you have relatives with these conditions.

Inform your healthcare supplier regarding your side effects so they can choose the best testing convention to decide out ailments that might be behind your weight loss battles.

12. Eat an entire foods-based eating routine

Perhaps the easiest approaches to guarantee that you give your body the supplements it needs to flourish is by following an eating routine wealthy in entire foods.

Entire foods, including vegetables, natural products, nuts, seeds, poultry, fish, vegetables, and grains, are pressed with supplements basic for keeping up healthy body wcight, for example, fibre, protein, and healthy fats.

Entire food-based eating regimens, both plant-based eating regimens and those that incorporate creature items, have been related to weight loss.

13. Eat less around evening time

Numerous researches have indicated that eating less calories around evening time may assist you with keeping up healthy body weight and lose abundance body fat.

Individuals who expended more calories can over multiple times bound to get large than individuals who ate more calories before in the day.

Individuals who have more calories at dinner were fundamentally bound to create metabolic disorder, a gathering of conditions including high glucose and abundance midsection fat. Metabolic disorder builds your danger of coronary illness, diabetes, and stroke.

Eating most of your calories during breakfast and lunch, while appreciating a lighter dinner, might be a beneficial technique to advance weight loss.

14. Concentrate on body organization

Despite the fact that bodyweight is a decent pointer of health, your body creation — which means the rates of fat and without fat mass in your body — is significant too.

Bulk is a significant proportion of overall health, particularly in more seasoned grown-ups. Pressing on more muscle and losing overabundance fat ought to be your objective

There are numerous approaches to quantify your body fat rate. In any case, just estimating your midsection, biceps, calves, chest, and thighs can assist you in deciding whether you're losing fat and picking up muscle.

15. Hydrate the healthy way

Beverages like improved espresso refreshments, pop, juices, sports drinks, and pre-made smoothies are regularly pressed with calories and included sugars.

Drinking sugar-improved refreshments, particularly those improved with high-fructose corn syrup, is firmly connected to weight addition and conditions like stoutness, coronary illness, diabetes, and fatty liver malady.

Swapping sugary refreshments with healthy beverages like water and natural tea can assist you with shedding pounds and may fundamentally reduce your danger of building up the incessant conditions referenced previously.

16. Pick the correct enhancements

On the off chance that you feel fatigued and unmotivated, taking the correct enhancements may help give you the vitality you have to arrive at your objectives.

As you become more seasoned, your capacity to retain certain supplements decreases, expanding your danger of inadequacies. For instance, explore shows that grown-ups over 50 are ordinarily inadequate in foliate and nutrient B12, two supplements that are required for vitality creation.

Lacks in B nutrients like B12 can contrarily affect your state of mind, cause fatigue, and impede weight loss.

Therefore, it's a smart thought for those over 50 to take a top-notch B-complex nutrient to help decline the danger of lack.

17. Farthest point included sugars

Constraining foods high in included sugar, including improved refreshments, treat, cakes, treats, dessert, improved yoghurts, and sugary grains, is basic for weight loss at any age.

Since sugar is added to such a significant number of foods, including things that you wouldn't expect like tomato sauce, a plate of mixed greens dressing, and bread, perusing fixing marks is the ideal approach to decide whether a thing contains included sugar.

Search for "included sugars" on the nourishment realities name or quest the fixing list for regular sugars, for example, genuine sweetener, high-fructose corn syrup, and agave.

18. Improve your rest quality

Not getting enough quality rest may hurt your weight loss endeavours. Numerous researchs have indicated that not getting enough rest improves the probability of stoutness and may thwart weight loss endeavours.

For instance, a 2-year study in 245 women showed that the individuals who rested 7 hours out of every night or more were 33% bound to shed pounds than women who dozed under 7 hours of the night. Better rest quality was likewise connected with weight loss achievement.

Intend to get the suggested 7–9 hours of rest for every night and improve your rest quality by limiting light in your room and avoiding utilizing your telephone or staring at the TV before bed.

19. Evaluate irregular fasting

Discontinuous fasting is a kind of eating design wherein you just eat during a predetermined period. The most well-known sort of irregular fasting is the 16/8 technique, where you eat inside an 8-hour window followed by a 16-hour quick.

Various researches have indicated that discontinuous fasting advances weight loss.

Furthermore, some test-cylinder and creature examine recommend that discontinuous fasting may profit more established grown-ups by expanding life span, easing back cell decay, and forestalling age-related changes to mitochondria, the vitality delivering portions of your phones.

20. Be increasingly careful

Careful eating can be a basic method to improve your association with food, all while encouraging weight loss.

Careful eating includes giving more consideration to your food and eating designs. It gives you a superior comprehension of your yearning and completion signs, just as how food impacts your mindset and prosperity.

Utilizing careful eating procedures advances weight loss and improves eating practices.

There are no particular principles to careful eating, yet eating gradually, focusing on the smell and kind of each nibble of food, and monitoring how you feel during your meals are basic approaches to acquaint careful eating with your life.

HEALTH BENEFITS OF KETO DIET FOR WOMEN OVER 50 YEARS

Benefits of the Ketogenic Diet for Women Over 50

"Eat healthier and get more exercise" is the go-to guide for pretty much any weight or health concern today. The inquiry is the thing that "eat healthier" signifies to every person. A great deal of that has to do with hormones, and maybe nobody realizes it superior to women over the age of 50.

One way of life change, specifically, is to present what is known as the Keto Diet. It's not so much an eating routine, yet a condition of the body, prompted by a protein-rich menu. What's more, it has someone of a kind highlights that are accounted for to affect health just like weight positively.

Fundamentally the same as the Atkins diet, many have utilized it to get thinner and make other health improvements just by confining the measure of carbohydrates in their eating routine.

Advantage #1: Fast Hassle-Free Weight Loss

As we age, our digestion normally eases back down around age 50, making it harder to get more fit. Perhaps the best advantage of the keto diet is that numerous individuals begin to shed pounds immediately. By limiting the measure of carbs taken in, our bodies would then be able to utilize fat stores for fuel.

At first, a great deal of water weight is lost, yet the uplifting news is, subsequent to moving beyond the main period of the eating routine our bodies modify. Sugar longings die down, vitality levels rise, and many even report more concentration and honed mental sharpness. There are no exacting point frameworks to follow or costly units to purchase. In the event that this arrangement sounds great to you, begin by loading up on explicit foods on your next basic food item run. Get things like:

- High protein meats like chicken, steak and seafood

- Breakfast foods, for example, wiener, bacon (indeed, bacon!!) and eggs.

- Full-fat dairy, for example, overwhelming cream and curds.

- Fresh spinach greens and non-boring vegetables

Advantage #2: Reportedly Helps Manage Type 2 Diabetes

For those determined to have diabetes or prediabetes in their 50s or 60s, the ketogenic diet may assist control with blooding glucose levels pushing ahead. As a result of the reduced sugar consumption, it's simpler for a body to manage blood glucose levels. This permits them to avoid sugar spikes and makes it simpler to create and control insulin levels.

Advantage #3: Combats Fatigue

Getting more seasoned and having more slow digestion regularly prompts feeling tired all the more frequently. A decent method to battle fatigue is to exercise and keep abundance weight off. With a keto benevolent eating regimen, you can nibble as much as you need (on the correct foods, obviously) without feeling hauled down in the wake of eating a meal. Being in a condition of ketosis, or fat-burning mode explicitly targets difficult midsection fat. Midsection fat prompts instinctive fat, which crushes inner organs and keeps them from working appropriately.

Advantage #4: Improves Neurological Health

Ageing can put us at an expanded hazard for dementia and certain types of it, for example, Alzheimer's malady. This could be on the grounds that an overload of glucose in the circulation system can make concentrating troublesome, which can influence your memory. Keeping levels relentless and in the typical range improves subjective capacity very quickly.

Weight gain is regular for some women in their 50s and past. The ketogenic might be a useful instrument to improve health and shed pounds as well! In the event that the aces exceed the cons in your book, converse with your PCP and check whether the keto diet is directly for you.

Advantage #5: Improves skin break out

Skin break out has a few distinct causes and may have connections to abstain from food and glucose in certain individuals. Eating an eating routine high in handled and refined carbohydrates may change the parity of gut microbes and cause glucose to rise and fall fundamentally, the two of which can unfavourably influence skin health.

Advantage #6: May reduce the danger of specific malignant growths

The ketogenic diet is forestalling or even treat certain diseases.

The ketogenic diet might be a sheltered and reasonable integral treatment to use close by chemotherapy and radiation treatment in individuals with specific malignancies. This is on the grounds that it would cause more oxidative worry in malignant growth cells than in ordinary cells, making them pass on.

The ketogenic diet reduces glucose. It could likewise bring down the danger of insulin inconveniences. Insulin is a hormone that controls glucose that may have connections to certain diseases.

Advantage #7: Potentially reduces seizures

The proportion of fat, protein, and carbs in a keto diet adjusts the manner in which the body utilizes vitality, bringing about ketosis. Ketosis is a metabolic procedure during which the body utilizes ketone bodies for fuel.

Ketosis can reduce seizures in individuals with epilepsy — particularly the individuals who have not reacted to other treatment techniques. Keto diet can bolster individuals with epilepsy. The ketogenic diet may reduce epilepsy side effects by a few unique components.

Advantage #8: Improves PCOS side effects

Polycystic ovary disorder (PCOS) is a hormonal issue that can prompt an abundance of male hormones, ovulatory brokenness, and polycystic ovaries. A high-starch diet can cause unfriendly impacts in individuals with PCOS, for example, skin problems and weight gain.

The ketogenic diet improved a few markers of PCOS, including:

- Weight loss

- Hormone balance

- Ratios of luteinizing hormone (LH) and follicle-animating hormone (FSH)

- Levels of fasting insulin

Keto diet had valuable impacts for individuals with hormonal disarranges, including PCOS and type 2 diabetes. Be that as it may, they did likewise alert that the investigations were too different even to consider recommending a keto diet as a general treatment for PCOS.

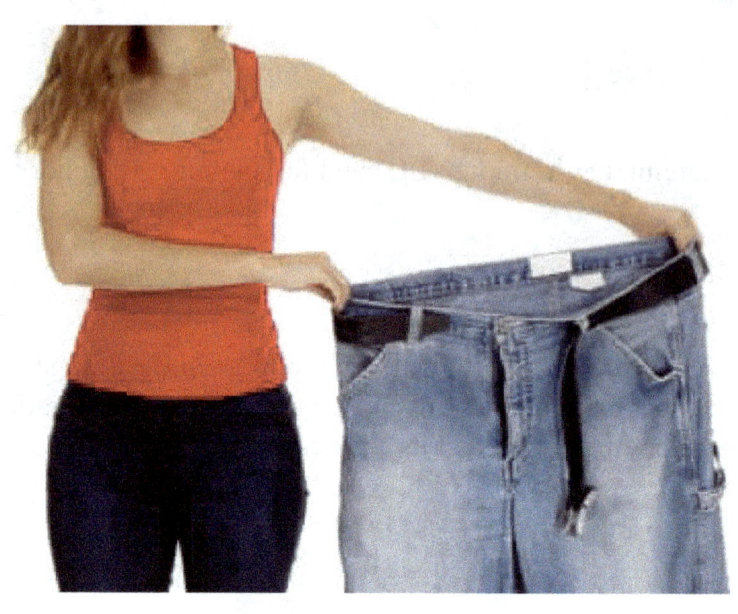

HOW TO GET KETOSIS

(FOOD CORRECT AND FOOD TO AVOID; HOW TO START; HOW TO MAKLE GRADUAL TRANSITION FROM A HIGH CARBOHYDRATES DIET)

INSTRUCTION TO GET INTO KETOSIS

7 tips to get into ketosis

Approaches to get the body into ketosis include:

1. Expanding physical action

An individual can get into ketosis by expanding physical action.

The more vitality that an individual uses during the day, the more food they have to eat for fuel.

Exercise enables an individual to drain the glycogen stores in their body. As a rule, the glycogen stores become renewed when an individual eats carbs. On the off chance that an individual is on a low-carb diet, they won't recharge their glycogen stores.

It can require some investment for the body to figure out how to utilize fat stores rather than glycogen. An individual may encounter fatigue as their body alters.

2. Essentially diminishing sugar consumption

Ketosis happens when an absence of starch powers the body to utilize fat as its essential vitality source rather than sugar.

An individual hoping to arrive at ketosis, regardless of whether for weight loss, to reduce the danger of coronary illness, or to keep up and control glucose levels, should mean to reduce their carb utilization to 20 grams (g) every day or less.

Notwithstanding, this is certifiably not a set number. A few people might have the option to eat more sugar and still get into a condition of ketosis, while others should eat less.

3. Fasting for brief periods

Fasting, or abandoning food, can enable an individual to accomplish a condition of ketosis. Numerous individuals can really go into ketosis between meals.

In some controlled cases, a specialist may prescribe a more drawn out fasting time of somewhere in the range of 24 and 48 hours. An individual ought to address their primary care physician before choosing to quick for longer than a couple of hours one after another.

Fat fasting is an elective type of fasting. Fat fasting includes fundamentally diminishing calorie admission and eating an eating regimen comprising for the most part of fat for close to 2 or 3 days.

This may positively affect weight loss. Nonetheless, fat fasting is hard to keep up and may not be the best alternative for a great many people.

Extremely little example sizes and the absence of progressively vigorous proof imply that individuals ought to be wary about adopting this strategy.

4. Expanding healthful fat admission

As sugar consumption diminishes, the vast majority supplant the loss of carbohydrates with an expansion in healthful fats. A few fats that an individual can eat include:

- coconut oil

- olive oil

- avocados and avocado oil

- flaxseed oil

Be that as it may, for individuals hoping to shed pounds, it is essential to remember the complete carbohydrate level also. Eating such a large number of calories in a day can make it harder to get more fit.

5. Testing ketone levels

One technique that can enable an individual to accomplish a condition of ketosis is observing the degrees of ketones in the body. There are a few tests accessible for this, including:

- urine

- breath

- blood

Utilizing at least one of these tests can enable an individual to keep tabs on their development, permitting them to make taught changes in accordance with their eating routine.

Ketone test strips are accessible to buy on the web.

6. Protein consumption

The keto diet confines the measure of protein an individual can eat in correlation with fat.

While suggested sums fluctuate, one standard keto diet prescribes expending 20% of calories as protein.

A low protein admission is essential for an individual to arrive at ketosis.

7. Devouring more coconut oil

Coconut oil may enable an individual to reach or keep up a condition of ketosis.

Adding coconut oil to the eating regimen may assist individuals with expanding their ketone levels.

Coconut oil contains fats called medium-chain triglycerides or MCTs. The body can retain MCTs rapidly and effectively. It at that point, sends these fats straightforwardly to the liver, which transforms them into either ketones or vitality.

Ketosis 5 Day Plan

DRINK WATER! You will know quickly however, that doesn't mean you're not going to drink water. You're going to drink a great deal of water. Keto is a characteristic diuretic – this implies you're going to pee a great deal. During the hours you're fasting you're likewise going to need to expand your salt admission. I like to utilize Ketone Salts.

At the point when you definitely reduce your carb consumption, your insulin-levels decline and your kidneys discharge more salt than when you were eating a lot of carbs. You're diminishing your insulin levels while getting into Ketosis (when you eat carbs, your insulin levels rise); salt isn't getting appropriately discharged by the body, and you're not ideally healthy. You rock, carbs! During this underlying stage, while getting into Ketosis, you must up the: Water, Calcium, and Magnesium, Sodium, and Potassium consumption. Normally, your salt cycle will reestablish, and your body is going to appropriately much obliged.

Day 0 - Sunday Night

•   Eat a Keto Dinner that is low in carbs (no later than 6pm).

•   Drink Water

•   Pee on a test strip (in case you're simply beginning, you're not going to change the shading on that little strip). Be that as it may, it's acceptable to see before you begin.

Day 1 - Monday

You're not going to eat food until 3pm. This is going to allow your body to free itself of however much of its Glycogen stores as could be expected. Holding off on eating until 3pm is a piece of this cleansing procedure (just piece of the procedure, however).

You're additionally going to need to get in (3) brief sessions of moderate/troublesome cardio. You're going to spread these brief sessions out (from when you wake up – till 3pm).

Suppose you wake up at 7am:

• Drink Water (with a spot of included, non-prepared genuine salt – no iodine) – Drink as much as you can. Keep it close by and promptly accessible – this applies for the duration of the day.

- 7:30 (10 Minutes of moderate/troublesome cardio)

- 10:00 (10 Minutes of moderate/troublesome cardio)

- 12:00 (Drink a serving of KetoCaNa or Ketone Salts)

- 12:15 (10 Minutes of moderate/troublesome cardio)

- 2:59 Pee on a test strip (in the event that you've spun through Ketosis previously, you may be in. If not, don't stress it's still early).

- 3:00 Eat a meal rich with dull verdant greens, fatty meat, avocados and healthy oils. Include a serving of MCT oil to whatever you're eating.

- You may eat Keto foods from 3pm – 8pm – Track your macros and feel full (don't overdo it).

- 8pm – It's water for you! Cheerful peeing.

- Before you hit the sack (1 serving of Magnesium)

- Pee on a test strip

You were simply acquainted with four enhancements. This is what they are:

- MCT Oil – Packed with nutritious fats, MCTs are consumed legitimately from the gut to the liver, where they are singed rapidly for vitality.

- KetoCaNa – KetoCaNa is a wellspring of ketones, giving 11.7 grams of BHB Salts per serving.

- Keto Salts – Calcium, Magnesium, Sodium, and Potassium (Ca, Ma, Na, K) – 13 Grams of Beta-Hydroxybutyrate Per Serving – Non-GMO, Gluten-Free, No Artificial Flavoring or Sweeteners

- Magnesium – Restores healthy magnesium levels and supports a healthy resistant framework. Magnesium advances typical circulatory strain and is required for delivering and putting away vitality.

Day 2 - Tuesday

Now (or yesterday evening after you ate) you might be feeling a touch of beating stomach, that is alright. In the event that you have a cerebral pain anytime make a point to expand your admission of water (with a touch of non-handled genuine salt).

Once more, we'll accept you woke up at 7 am.

- Pee on a test strip

- Drink Water

- 12:00 (Drink a serving of KetoCaNa or Ketone Salts)

- 12:15 (10 Minutes of moderate/troublesome cardio)

- 12:59 Pee on a test strip

- 1:00 Lunch Time! Eat a meal rich with dull verdant greens and fatty meat. Look at our Keto recipes for thoughts on what to eat. Include a serving of MCT oil to whatever you're eating.

- You may eat Keto foods from 1 pm – 8 pm – Track your macros and feel full (don't overdo it).

- 8 pm – It's water for you! Glad peeing.

- Before you hit the hay (1 serving of Magnesium)

- Pee on a test strip

Day 3 - Wednesday

Wednesday will be a similar procedure as Tuesday, and you very may well as of now be in Ketosis! Be that as it may, on the off chance that you are not, here is the convention to follow:

Once more, we'll expect you woke up at 7 am.

- Pee on a test strip

- Drink Water

- 12:00 (Drink a serving of KetoCaNa or Ketone Salts)

- 12:15 (10 Minutes of moderate/troublesome cardio)

- 12:59 Pee on a test strip

- 1:00 Lunch Time! Eat a meal rich with dim verdant greens and fatty meat. Look at our Keto recipes for thoughts on what to eat. Include a serving of MCT oil to whatever you're eating.

- You may eat Keto foods from 1 pm – 8 pm – Track your macros and feel full (don't overdo it).

- 8 pm – It's water for you! Glad peeing.

- Before you hit the sack (1 serving of Magnesium)

- Pee on a test strip

Day 4 - Thursday

Your body should as of now be in ketosis, yet in the event that it's not, you will be following a similar custom as you did on Day 2:

Once more, we'll expect you woke up at 7 am.

- Pee on a test strip

- Drink Water

- 12:00 (Drink a serving of KetoCaNa or Ketone Salts)

- 12:15 (10 Minutes of moderate/troublesome cardio)

- 12:59 Pee on a test strip

- 1:00 Lunch Time! Eat a meal rich with dim verdant greens and fatty meat. Look at our Keto recipes for thoughts on what to eat. Include a serving of MCT oil to whatever you're eating.

- You may eat Keto foods from 1 pm – 8 pm – Track your macros and feel full (don't overdo it).

- 8 pm – It's water for you! Cheerful peeing.

- Before you hit the sack (1 serving of Magnesium)

- Pee on a test strip

Day 5+

Congrats! You ought to be in ketosis, and would now be able to follow an ordinary keto meal intend to stay with it.

FOOD TO EAT AND FOODD TO AVOID FOR WOMEN OVER 50

While the nature of your eating regimen can influence your health at any age, keeping up a healthy way of life and eating clean is significantly progressively significant after age 50. A lot of ceaseless and genuine maladies, from malignant growth to coronary illness, become increasingly pervasive when you're 50+, and eating right can help alleviate your risks — in addition, give you the vitality to need to remain dynamic and healthy well past middle age. Eating healthy after 50 doesn't need to be troublesome, either. Simply remember these healthy foods for your eating regimen to get the supplements you need, and avoid foods that will destroy your vitality and add to the ageing procedure.

- Flaxseed. Flaxseeds have antioxidants. ...

- Unsweetened almond milk. Go for unsweetened almond milk. ...

- Cinnamon. Cinnamon can help battle against diabetes. ...

- Eggs. Eggs bolster a healthy immune framework. ...

- Potatoes. Potatoes are extremely healthy … simply don't sear them. ...

- Wild Alaskan salmon. ...

- Tempeh. ...

- Beans.

- salom

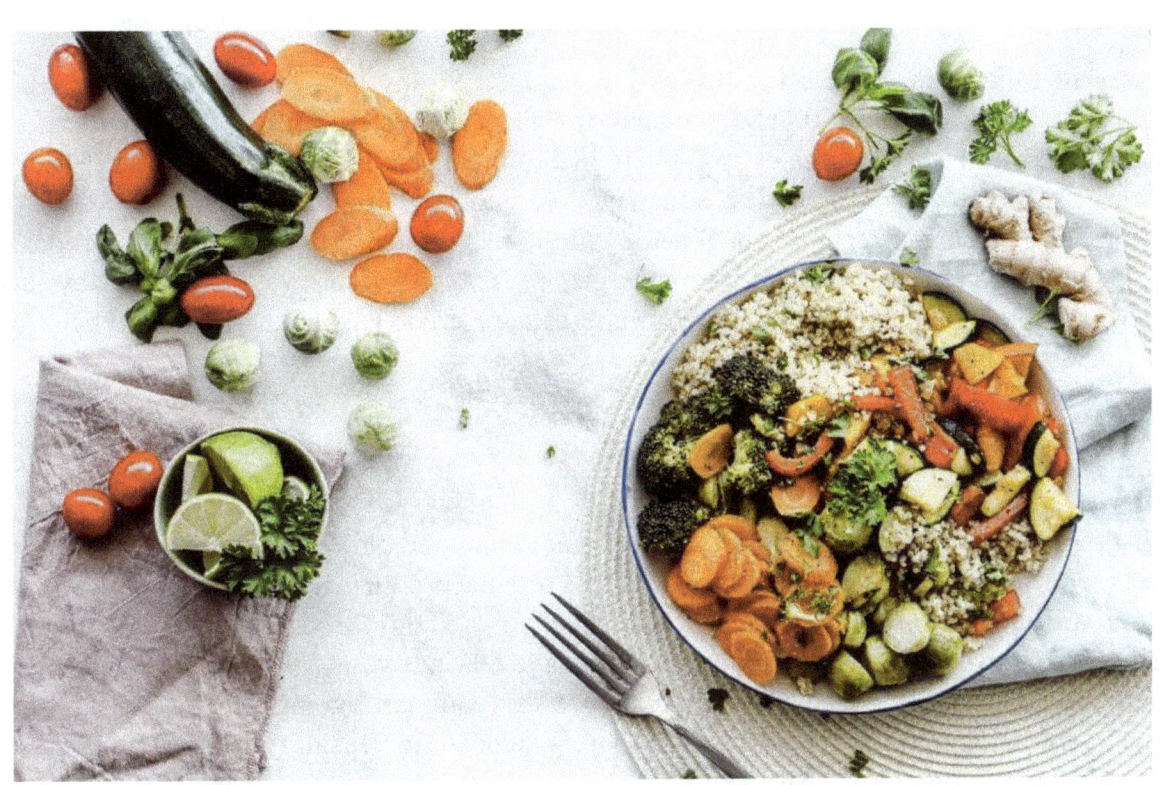

Foods to Eat: Broccoli, Spinach and Kale

Veggies are a basic piece of a healthy eating regimen at any age, yet these three greens are particularly significant after 50. The explanation? They're pressed with two carotenoids, called lutein and zeaxanthin. This force couple offers incredible insurance for your eyes since they help to channel the blue light that maybe some way or another harm your retinas and add to eye infections like macular degeneration. Since eye ailments regularly grow further down the road, center on getting a greater amount of these veggies presently to secure your peepers. Have a go at simmering broccoli with garlic and lemon or appreciate a crude kale plate of mixed greens hurled with crimson oranges.

Citrus Fruits

A half-grapefruit in the first part of the day may feel like good old eating routine food. However, it merits returning to this healthy exemplary. Citrus organic products like grapefruit, orange, lemon and lime all huge inventory amounts of nutrient C. Your body needs nutrient C to create new collagen — and that is particularly significant after age 50 since your collagen will work in general separate all the more rapidly as a component of the common ageing procedure. Keeping up collagen generation not just keeps you skin more grounded, increasingly versatile and energetic, yet in addition reinforces your hair, veins, joints and other connective tissues.

SALOM

Fatty fish like wild salmon, mackerel, and herring owe their super health-elevating forces to their high omega-3 substance. These incredible anti-provocative fatty acids can help decline your chances of biting the dust from coronary illness by in excess of 33 per cent, help bring down your danger of joint pain, and conceivably make your infant more astute. To see which omega-3 fish you ought to bring, within proper limits out our restrictive report of fish positioned for dietary benefits.

Pecans

Securing your most fundamental organ is as straightforward as adding a few pecans to your eating regimen. This heart-formed nut is overflowing with antioxidants and omega-3 fatty acids that can help guard you.

Grown Garlic

About 33% of women somewhere in the range of 45 and 55 have hypertension, an illness that can prompt increasingly major issues like coronary illness or stroke, and that number increments from 50 to 70 per cent for women matured 55 to those 65 and more established. It turns out; the vampire-repulsing plant is both a flavour basic and a coronary illness battling hotshot. Garlic contains phytochemicals, including allicin, Garlic can likewise forestall the movement of coronary illness by lessening the gathering of plaque and forestalling the development of new plaque in the conduits.

Apples

Perhaps the best food women ought to eat is one you presumably as of now are: the apple. Metabolic disorder—a disorder that alludes to a group of conditions like insulin obstruction, hypertension, and elevated cholesterol—is the primary supporter of coronary illness, the main enemy of American women. While women who eat an eating regimen wealthy in glucose spiking refined carbs or the individuals who are overweight are generally defenceless to a metabolic disorder, even healthy postmenopausal women are likewise in danger.

Beans

In contrast to creature wellsprings of protein, beans are liberated from unhealthy fats.

Eating a 3/4 of a cup of beans day by day could reduce levels of "terrible" cholesterol in the blood by 5 per cent.

Shrimp

Shrimp is the most powerful wellspring of a fundamental and difficult-to-get supplement called choline. This synapse building square is essential for the structure and capacity of all things considered, and a lack right now been connected to neurological clutters and diminished psychological capacity. In addition to the fact that it acts as mind food, yet it can likewise help bring down your danger of bosom malignancy.

Blueberries

Blueberries are one of the most intense, age-resisting, antioxidant-rich superfoods. Their wide cluster of health benefits is, for the most part, ascribed to their incredible anthocyanins, antioxidants, which wash down your body of cell-damaging free radicals.

These equivalent antioxidants that help keep up your psychological sharpness additionally help keep your skin smooth and without wrinkle—something each lady would be enthusiastic about. Yet, that is not every one of; these organic products help battle coronary illness alongside other berry benefits.

Almond Butter

Swapping nutty spread for almond margarine may better your odds of beating age-related memory loss. Almonds contain high convergences of nutrient E (multiple times more than nutty spread), which has been appeared to help reduce the danger of subjective impedance.

Turmeric

Bosom malignant growth is the most well-known disease in women worldwide and the subsequent driving reason for disease-related mortality in women.

One approach to reducing the mortality of disease is through prevention, and that can be practised by eating turmeric. This ginger-family flavour contains curcumin, an antioxidant polyphenol with chemopreventive properties. Ceaseless aggravation is a significant hazard factor for the development and metastatic movement of malignant growth, and curcumin's anti-incendiary properties have been found to reduce the arrangement of bosom disease.

Tomatoes

Tomatoes can help shield our DNA from harm that can prompt bosom, endometrial, lung, stomach, prostate, and renal cell carcinoma malignant growths,

Warming procedure expands the measure of lycopene that is accessible for your body to ingest, ensure you include tomato glue, sautéed tomatoes, or a natural tomato sauce to omelettes, chicken and pasta dishes to receive the rewards.

Pomegranate

Pomegranates have been connected to ripeness and health for a considerable length of time; however today, specialists are captivated with the seeded organic product's capacity to restrain the development of the hormone-subordinate bosom disease.

Portabella Mushrooms

In addition to the fact that mushrooms are excessively low-cal, they're a decent wellspring of potassium, a supplement that can assist lower with blooding weight and balance the negative impacts of abundance sodium. Another motivation to add the veggie to your shopping list:

Specialists ascribe the expansion to mushrooms' significant levels of nutrient D, and portobello mushrooms brag the best fixation.

Olive Oil and Fatty Fish

Healthy fats advantage individuals everything being equal since the fat in your food makes certain supplements simpler to retain and secures against supplement lacks. Yet, picking the correct fats is particularly significant as you age, since you face a greater danger of creating cardiovascular illness than you did in your childhood. The unsaturated fats found in olive oil and fatty fish (like salmon, sardines and fish) help deal with your blood cholesterol. Joined with an overall healthy eating routine and way of life, they can help keep your coronary illness chance as low as could be expected under the circumstances. Add salmon to your eating regimen by either heating it, container searing or barbecuing it.

Heartbeats

With regards to healthy eating, beats — lentils, beans and peas — are about at least somewhat great. A triple risk, beats are incredibly low in cost (think pennies per serving!), and they're stacked with filling fibre and protein. Likewise important: they have a low vitality thickness, which implies they keep up a moderately low carbohydrate level in spite of a liberal and filling serving size. Eating low vitality thickness foods turns out to be increasingly more significant as you age since your digestion can back off and trigger unexpected weight gain. Remembering more heartbeats for your eating regimen makes it simpler to get control over your calorie admission without feeling denied. Here's the way to appropriately cook lentils.

Quinoa, Barley and Other Whole Grains

In the event that you haven't made a propensity for eating entire grains, it's an ideal opportunity to begin. Not exclusively do entire grains offer more surface, which can cause your food to feel all the more filling, but on the other hand, they're an extraordinary wellspring of dietary fibre. Getting enough fibre is fundamental for staying, um, normal — yet fibre additionally helps bring down the danger of stomach related clutters like diverticulitis, which will, in general, be increasingly regular in more established grown-ups. Get entire grain toast, serve dark coloured or wild rice as a staple side dish, or appreciate a healthy dish of a wild mushroom quinoa risotto.

FOOD TO AVOID FOR WOMEN OVER 50

- Pickles. Bid farewell to this salty tidbit. ...

- Potatoes. Just eat these every so often. ...

- Breakfast cakes. The outcomes may not be justified, despite all the trouble. ...

- Butter. Attempt olive oil. ...

- Too much wine. Keep in mind everything with some restraint. ...

- Deli meats. Prepared meats are high in salt and fat. ...

-     Steam pack solidified vegetables. ...

-     Deep dish pizza.

Food to Avoid: Sugary Smoothies

Spinach and kale are regularly connected with smoothies these days — yet in case you're presenting that veggie smoothie with bunches of included sugar (or nectar, or maple syrup, or agave...) you should reconsider your decision. Improved smoothies can rapidly pile on handfuls or even several calories from sugar. Not exclusively can all that sugar add to weight gain, yet it can likewise make it hard to control your blood glucose levels — and constantly high glucose can harm your eyes, kidneys and different tissues. Improve your smoothies with a half-cup to a cup of organic product. Over time, your sense of taste will acclimate to the absence of sugar.

Seared Foods

Also, on the opposite finish of the anti-ageing range, we have seared foods — one of the most exceedingly terrible things you can eat in case you're attempting to remain energetic. Seared and fatty foods are stuffed with calories, thanks to a limited extent to all the fat they contain. Separating the fat makes responsive mixes, called free radicals, that can possibly harm your phones and quicken the ageing procedure. Obviously, seared foods have different disadvantages also, from adding to diabetes and weight to expanding your danger of cardiovascular illness. Simply state, no!

Margarine

When thought of as a healthier choice to spread, margarine should now top your "Don't BUY" list. That is on the grounds that creating a few kinds of margarine includes a procedure called hydrogenation, during which the fats experience a compound change that diverts them from fluids at room temperature into solids. Hydrogenated fats are additionally called trans fats, and they're the most exceedingly terrible fat you can eat with regards to raising your coronary illness chance.

Granola

Also, on the opposite finish of the range, we have granola. While granola may sound healthy — all things considered, it's simply oats, nuts and organic product — it has incredibly high vitality thickness. Indeed, a quarter-cup serving of economically accessible granola has 120 calories... what's more, who eats only a quarter-cup, in any case? Foods with a high vitality thickness are bound to make you put on weight since they pack heaps of calories into a little serving. Also, you're increasingly more prone to gain weight as you age and your digestion eases back down. In the event that you love granola, attempt muesli rather — you'll get a comparative preference for less calories.

Refined Grains and Flour

Changing to entire grain implies removing refined (white) grains and flour — and that is something worth being thankful for, on the grounds that these foods fail to help you. While refined grains are stuffed with calories, they come up short on the fibre that would somehow or another cause you to feel full. An eating regimen high in refined grains likewise raises your danger of type 2 diabetes and coronary illness — ailments that you're as of now confronting a greater danger old enough you age. It might be difficult to reset your sense of taste to acknowledge entire grains when you're utilized to refined ones. However, it merits the push to discard whatever number of these handled grains as could reasonably be expected.

HOW TO MAKE GRADUAL TRANSITION FROM A HIGH CARB DIET

Decreasing carbohydrates can have significant benefits for your health.

Low-carb diets can assist you in getting more fit and control diabetes or prediabetes.

Here are 15 simple approaches to reduce your carb consumption.

1. Wipeout Sugar-Sweetened Drinks

Sugar-improved drinks are unhealthy.

They're high in included sugar, which is connected to an expanded danger of insulin obstruction, type 2 diabetes and heftiness when expended in overabundance.

A 12-ounce (354-ml) container of sugary soft drink contains 38 grams of carbs, and a 12-ounce improved frosted tea has 36 grams of carbs. These come totally from sugar.

On the off chance that you need to eat less carbs, avoiding sugar-improved refreshments ought to be one of the principal things you do.

On the off chance that you need to drink something invigorating with a taste, have a go at adding some lemon or lime to club pop or frosted tea. If necessary, utilize a limited quantity of low-calorie sugar.

2. Cut Back on Bread

Bread is a staple food in numerous eating regimens. Sadly, it's additionally very high in carbs and by and large low in fibre.

This is particularly valid for white bread produced using refined grains, which may contrarily affect health and weight.

Indeed, even nutritious bread, for example, rye contains around 15 grams of carbs per cut. What's more, just a few those are fibre, the main segment of carbs that aren't processed and retained.

Albeit entire grain bread contains nutrients and minerals, there are numerous different foods that furnish similar supplements with many less carbs.

These healthy foods incorporate vegetables, nuts and seeds.

In any case, it very well may be difficult to surrender bread totally. In case you think that it's troublesome, attempt one of these flavorful low-carb bread recipes that are anything but difficult to make.

Entire grain bread contains some significant supplements. However, these can be found in numerous different foods that are lower in carbs.

3. Quit Drinking Fruit Juice

In contrast to the entire organic product, natural product juice contains practically zero fibre and is brimming with sugar.

In spite of the fact that it gives a few nutrients and minerals, it's no superior to sugar-improved refreshments as far as sugar and carbs. This is genuine in any event, for 100% organic product juice.

For example, 12 oz (354 ml) of 100% squeezed apple contains 48 grams of carbs, the greater part of which is sugar.

It's ideal to avoid squeeze totally. Rather, take a stab at seasoning your water by including a cut of orange or lemon.

Organic product juice contains the same number of carbs as sugar-improved drinks. Rather than drinking juice, include a modest quantity of natural product to water.

4. Pick Low-Carb Snacks

Carbs can include rapidly in nibble foods, for example, chips, pretzels and wafers.

These kinds of foods are, likewise, not very satisfying. Women felt more full and ate 100 less calories at dinner when they ate a high-protein nibble, contrasted with a low-protein one.

Having a low-carb bite that contains protein is the best system when the craving strikes between meals.

Here are a couple of healthy tidbits that contain under 5 grams of edible (net) carbs per 1-oz (28-gram) serving and furthermore some protein:

- Almonds: 6 grams of carbs, 3 of which are fibre.

- Peanuts: 6 grams of carbs, 2 of which are fibre.

- Macadamia nuts: 4 grams of carbs, 2 of which are fibre.

- Hazelnuts: 5 grams of carbs, 3 of which are fibre.

- Pecans: 4 grams of carbs, 3 of which are fibre.

- Walnuts: 4 grams of carbs, 2 of which are fibre.

- Cheese: Less than 1 gram of carbs.

Make a point to have healthy low-carb snacks, for example, nuts and cheddar available in the event that you get ravenous between meals.

5. Eat Eggs or Other Low-Carb Breakfast Foods

Indeed, even modest quantities of some morning meal foods are regularly high in carbs.

For example, one half-cup (55 grams) of granola oat normally has around 30 grams of absorbable carbs, even before including milk.

On the other hand, eggs are a perfect breakfast when you're attempting to reduce carbs.

First of all, each egg contains under 1 gram of carbs. They're additionally an incredible wellspring of top-notch protein, which can assist you with feeling full for quite a long time and eat less calories during the remainder of the day.

Likewise, eggs are amazingly flexible and can be set up from numerous points of view, remembering hard-bubbling for a for the-go breakfast.

For breakfast recipes highlighting eggs and other low-carb foods

Picking eggs or other high-protein, low-carb foods for breakfast can assist you with feeling full and fulfilled for a few hours.

6. Utilize These Sweeteners Instead of Sugar

Utilizing sugar to improve foods and drinks is definitely not a healthy practice, especially on a low-carb diet.

One tablespoon of white or dark coloured sugar has 12 grams of carbs as sucrose, which is 50% fructose and 50% glucose

Albeit nectar may appear to be healthier, it's considerably higher in carbs. One tablespoon gives 17 grams of carbs, with generally a similar level of fructose and glucose as sugar.

Figuring out how to appreciate the common kind of foods without including any sugar may, at last, be ideal.

Be that as it may, here are a couple of safe without sugar sugars that may even have some unobtrusive health benefits:

- Erythritol: Erythritol is a sort of sugar liquor that has an aftertaste like sugar, doesn't raise glucose or insulin levels and may help forestall depressions by murdering plaque-causing microbes

- Xylitol: Another sugar liquor, xylitol likewise helps battle the microbes that cause tooth rot. What's more, creature explore proposes it might reduce insulin opposition and ensure against obesitY.

Utilizing low-calorie sugar options can assist you with keeping your carb admission low without surrendering sweetness through and through.

7. Request Veggies Instead of Potatoes or Bread at Restaurants

Eating out can be trying during the underlying phases of a low-carb diet.

Regardless of whether you request meat or fish with no breading or sauce, you'll normally get a starch as an afterthought. This is regularly potatoes, pasta, bread or rolls.

In any case, these starches can add 30 grams of carbs to your meal or more. It relies upon the part size, which is regularly very huge.

Rather, request that your server substitute low-carb vegetables instead of the high-carb foods. In the event that your meal as of now incorporates a side of vegetables, you can have another serving, as long as the vegetables are the non-dull sort.

Getting vegetables rather than potatoes, pasta or bread when eating out can spare numerous carbs.

8. Substitute Low-Carb Flours for Wheat Flour

Wheat flour is a high-carb fixing in most prepared merchandise, including bread, biscuits and treats. It's likewise utilized for covering meat and fish preceding sauteing or heating.

Indeed, even entire wheat flour, which contains more fibre than refined white flour, has 61 grams of absorbable carbs per 100 grams (3.5 ounces)

Luckily, flours produced using nuts and coconuts are an incredible other option and generally accessible at markets and from online retailers.

100 grams of almond flour contains under 11 grams of edible carbs, and 100 grams of coconut flour contains 21 grams of edible carbs

These flours can be utilized to cover foods for sautéing, just as in recipes that call for wheat flour. Notwithstanding, in light of the fact that they don't contain gluten, the surface of the completed item frequently won't be the equivalent.

Almond and coconut flour will in general work best in recipes for biscuits, hotcakes and comparative delicate, prepared products.

Use almond or coconut flour instead of wheat flour in heated products or when covering food before sauteing or preparing.

9. Supplant Milk with Almond or Coconut Milk

Milk is nutritious, but at the same time, it's genuinely high in carbs in light of the fact that it contains a kind of sugar called lactose.

An 8-ounce (240 ml) glass of full-fat or low-fat milk contains 12–13 grams of carbs

Adding a sprinkle of milk to your espresso or tea is fine.

However, in the event that you drink milk by the glassful or in lattes or shakes, it might wind up contributing a lot of carbs

There are a few milk substitutes accessible. The most mainstreams are coconut and almond milk. However, there are additional types produced using different nuts and hemp. Nutrient D, calcium and different nutrients and minerals are regularly added to improve healthy benefit.

These refreshments are chiefly water, and the carb content is normally low. Most have 2 grams of absorbable carbs or less per serving.

Notwithstanding, some contain sugar, so make certain to check the fixing rundown and nourishment name to ensure you're getting an unsweetened, low-carb refreshment.

Use almond milk, coconut milk or other elective low-carb milk substitutes instead of customary milk.

10. Accentuate Non-Starchy Veggies

Vegetables are an important wellspring of supplements and fibre on a low-carb diet. They additionally contain phytochemicals (plant mixes), a significant number of which work as antioxidants that help shield you from illness

Nonetheless, it's critical to choose non-boring sorts to keep your carb consumption down.

Certain root vegetables and vegetables, for example, carrots, beets, sweet potatoes, peas, lima beans and corn, are decently high in carbs.

Luckily, there are numerous delightful, feeding low-carb veggies you can eat.

Pick non-bland vegetables to keep your carb consumption low while keeping up a high admission of supplements and fibre.

11. Pick Dairy That is Low in Carbs

Dairy items are tasty and can be exceptionally healthy. First of all, they contain calcium, magnesium and other significant minerals.

Dairy additionally contains conjugated linoleic corrosive (CLA), a sort of fatty corrosive which has been appeared to advance fat loss in a few researches.

Notwithstanding, some dairy foods are terrible decisions on a low-carb diet. For example, natural product seasoned yoghurt, solidified yoghurt and pudding are frequently stacked with sugar and extremely high in carbs.

Then again, Greek yoghurt and cheddar are a lot of lower in carbs and have been appeared to reduce craving, advance totality, improve body creation and reduce coronary illness chance elements.

Here are a couple of good dairy decisions, alongside carb tallies per 100 grams (3.5 oz):

- Plain Greek yoghurt: 4 grams of carbs.

- Cheese (brie, mozzarella, cheddar, and so on.): 1 gram of carbs.

- Ricotta cheddar: 3 grams of carbs.

- Cottage cheddar: 3 grams of carbs.

Pick Greek yoghurt and cheddar so as to acquire the benefits of dairy with not very many carbs.

12. Eat Healthy High-Protein Foods

Eating a decent protein source at each meal can make it simpler to decrease carbs, and it's especially significant in case you're attempting to get more fit.

Protein triggers the arrival of the "completion hormone" PYY, reduces hunger, helps battle food longings and ensures bulk during weight loss.

Protein additionally has a lot higher thermic worth contrasted with fat or carbs, which means your body's metabolic rate builds more while processing and using it

Make a point to incorporate in any event one serving from this rundown of high-protein, low-carb foods at every meal:

- Meat
- Poultry

- Fish

- Eggs

- Nuts

- Cheese

- Cottage cheddar

- Greek yoghurt

- Whey protein powder

- Consuming healthy protein at each meal can assist you with feeling full, battle desires and lift your metabolic rate.

13. Get ready Foods with Healthy Fats

Fat replaces some carbs and commonly makes up over 50% of calories on a low-carb diet.

In this manner, it's imperative to pick fats that include season as well as advantage your health. Two of the healthiest decisions are virgin coconut oil and extra-virgin olive oil.

Virgin coconut oil is a profoundly soaked fat that is truly steady at high cooking temperatures. A large portion of its fat is medium-chain triglycerides (MCTs), which may reduce tummy fat and increment HDL cholesterol.

Furthermore, these MCTs may likewise diminish hunger. In one research, men who had an MCT-rich breakfast ate fundamentally less calories at lunch than men who had a morning meal high in long-chain triglycerides

Extra-virgin olive oil has been appeared to reduce circulatory strain, improve the capacity of the cells covering your conduits and help forestall weight gain.

Planning low-carb foods with healthy fats can upgrade enhance, advance sentiments of totality and improve your health.

14. Begin Reading Food Labels

Seeing food names can give important data about the carb substance of bundled foods.

The key is realizing where to look and whether any estimations should be finished. In the event that you live outside the US, the fibre in the carbs area will have just been deducted.

In the event that you live in the US, you can deduct the grams of fibre from the carbs to get the edible ("net") carb content.

It's likewise critical to take a gander at what number of servings are remembered for the bundle, as it's frequently more than one.

In the event that a path blend contains 7 grams of carbs per serving and an aggregate of 4 servings, you'll wind up taking in 28 grams of carbs on the off chance that you eat the entire pack.

Perusing food names can assist you in deciding what number of carbs are in bundled foods.

15. Check Carbs With a Nutrition Tracker

A nourishment tracker is a great apparatus for monitoring your day by day food consumption. Most are accessible as applications for cell phones and tablets, just as on the web.

At the point when you enter your food consumption for every meal and nibble, carbs and different supplements are naturally determined.

These projects ascertain your supplement needs dependent on your weight, age and different elements. However, you can tweak your day by day carb objective and change it when you like.

The vast majority of the data in the food databases is reliable. In any case, remember that a portion of these projects permits individuals to include custom sustenance data that may not generally be exact.

Utilizing sustenance following application or online program can assist you with observing and adjust your carb admission.

HOW TO AVOID KETO FLU FOR OVER 50

Keto influenza is an assortment of side effects experienced by certain individuals when they are first beginning the keto diet.

These manifestations, which can feel like this season's cold virus, are brought about by the body adjusting to another eating regimen comprising of next to no carbohydrates.

Diminishing your carb consumption powers your body to consume ketones for vitality rather than glucose.

Ketones are side-effects of fat breakdown and become the primary fuel source when following a ketogenic diet.

Regularly, fat is saved as an auxiliary fuel source to utilize when glucose isn't accessible. This change to burning fat for vitality is called ketosis. It happens during explicit conditions, including starvation and fasting.

In any case, ketosis can likewise be come to by embracing a low-carb diet.

In a ketogenic diet, carbohydrates are normally reduced to under 50 grams every day.

This radical decrease can come as a stun to the body and may cause withdrawal-like manifestations, like those accomplished when weaning off an addictive substance like caffeine.

Keto influenza is a term used to portray influenza-like side effects related to starting the low-carb ketogenic diet.

Keto influenza can cause you to feel hopeless.

Fortunately, there are approaches to reduce its influenza-like side effects and help your body traverse the change time frame all the more effectively.

APPROACHES TO GET RID OF KETO FLU FOR WOMEN OVER 50

Remain Hydrated

Drinking enough water is vital for ideal health and can likewise help reduce manifestations.

A keto diet can make you quickly shed water stores, expanding the danger of parchedness.

This is on the grounds that glycogen, the put-away type of carbohydrates, ties to water in the body. At the point when dietary carbohydrates are reduced, glycogen levels fall, and water is discharged from the body.

Remaining hydrated can help with manifestations like fatigue and muscle squeezing.

Supplanting liquids is particularly significant when you are encountering keto-influenza related looseness of the bowels, which can cause extra liquid loss.

Avoid Strenuous Exercise

While exercise is significant for remaining healthy and holding body weight in line, strenuous exercise ought to be avoided while encountering keto-influenza manifestations.

Fatigue, muscle issues and stomach uneasiness are normal in the main seven day stretch of following a ketogenic diet, so it might be a smart thought to give your body a rest.

Exercises like extraordinary biking, running, weight lifting and strenuous exercises may be set aside for later while your framework adjusts to new fuel sources.

While these kinds of exercise ought to be avoided on the off chance that you are encountering the keto influenza, light exercises like strolling, yoga or restful biking may improve manifestations.

Get an influenza shot.

Getting an influenza shot is the absolute best thing that you can do every influenza season to shield yourself from extreme illness.

An influenza shot offers the best insurance from influenza infections.

Occasional influenza shots — made to secure against three or four influenza infections that are accepted to be the most well-known during a particular influenza season — are antibodies that are typically infused into the arm with a needle.

Influenza immunizations trigger antibodies to create in the body, for the most part inside about fourteen days of having a shot. The antibodies give insurance against the strains of influenza contamination contained in the immunization. In spite of the fact that this season's cold virus shot may have symptoms in certain individuals, it can't cause influenza illness.

Influenza shot diminished the probability of inconveniences and demise — in any event when contamination neglects to be forestalled.

Who ought to get this season's cold virus shot?

Everybody over the age of a half year is prescribed to get a yearly influenza inoculation, as per the Centers for Disease Control and Prevention (CDC). A few influenza shots are accessible, relying upon age and whether you are pregnant or have a constant health condition.

Kids under a half-year-old are too youthful even to consider receiving an influenza shot. Individuals who have dangerous hypersensitivities to any fixing in the antibody or have ever had Guillain-Barré disorder ought to examine this season's flu virus shot with their primary care physician before getting immunized.

At the point when the stockpile of the antibody is restricted, need will frequently be given to:

- children matured between a half year and 4 years
- adults matured 50 years and over
- those with a constant pneumonic issue or who are immunosuppressed
- pregnant women
- children and youths on long haul headache medicine treatment
- people who work in constant consideration offices and healthcare faculty
- individuals with a body mass list (BMI) of at least 40

In individuals in danger of coronary illness, their danger of cardiovascular failure is multiple times higher in the initial 7 days of influenza.

Supplant Electrolytes

Supplanting dietary electrolytes may help reduce keto-influenza side effects.

When following a ketogenic diet, levels of insulin, a significant hormone that enables the body to assimilate glucose from the circulatory system, decline.

At the point when insulin levels decline, the kidneys discharge overabundance sodium from the body.

Furthermore, the keto diet limits numerous foods that are high in potassium, including natural products, beans and boring vegetables.

Getting sufficient measures of these significant supplements is a great method to control through the adjustment time of the eating regimen.

Salting food to taste and including potassium-rich, keto-accommodating foods like green verdant vegetables and avocados are a phenomenal method to guarantee you are keeping up a healthy equalization of electrolytes.

These foods are likewise high in magnesium, which may help reduce muscle cramps, rest issues and migraines.

Get Adequate Sleep

Fatigue and peevishness are basic grumblings of individuals who are adjusting to a ketogenic diet.

Absence of rest causes levels of the pressure hormone cortisol to ascend in the body, which can adversely affect mind-set and aggravate keto-influenza side effects.

In the event that you are making some troublesome memories falling or staying unconscious, attempt one of the accompanying tips:

- Reduce caffeine consumption: Caffeine is an energizer that may adversely affect rest. In the event that you drink juiced refreshments, just do as such in the first part of the day, so your rest isn't influenced.

- Cut out encompassing light: Shut off phones, PCs and TVs in the room to make a dim domain and advance relaxing rest.

- Take a shower: Adding Epsom salt or basic lavender oil to your shower is a loosening up approach to slow down and prepare for rest.

- Get up ahead of schedule: Waking simultaneously consistently and avoiding oversleeping may help standardize your rest designs and improve rest quality over time.

Ensure You Are Eating Enough Fat (and Carbs)

Changing to a low-carb diet can make you ache for foods that are confined on the ketogenic diet, for example, treats, bread, pasta and bagels.

Be that as it may, eating enough fat, the essential fuel source on the ketogenic diet, will help reduce yearnings and keep you feeling fulfilled.

Truth be told, examine shows that low-carb counts calories help reduce yearnings for desserts and high-carb foods.

Those making some troublesome memories adjusting to the ketogenic diet may need to wipe out carbohydrates continuously, as opposed to at the same time.

Gradually curtailing carbs, while expanding fat and protein in your eating routine, may help make the change smoother and abatement keto-influenza side effects.

You can battle the keto influenza by remaining hydrated, supplanting electrolytes, getting a lot of rest, avoiding strenuous exercises, eating enough fat and removing carbs gradually over time.

Adjusting to the ketogenic diet can feel like this season's cold virus. Tiredness, fatigue, stomach torments, and discombobulating are normal side effects that the ketogenic diet apprentice can understanding. However, these manifestations don't originate from a ketogenic infection or a tainted mosketo (like "mosquito")

Actually, the side effects for keto influenza are not brought about by ketosis, ketogenesis, or this season's cold virus by any means. Keto influenza is brought about by the body's reaction to sugar limitation.

TIPS AND TRICKS ON KETOGENIC DIET FOR WOMEN ABOVE 50

#1: Try Intermittent Fasting

Discontinuous fasting (IF) is apparently the best tip for women over 50 can place enthusiastically immediately to get into ketosis and assist you with getting more fit — if that is the objective.

This means you don't eat or drink whatever contains calories for a distributed timeframe.

Discontinuous fasting can control your body's mitochondria in comparative manners as the ketogenic diet to build your life expectancy and furthermore makes you look more youthful than your age.

At the point when you don't expend calories for a couple of hours, your body begins exhausting the entirety of the overabundance glucose that is put away in your body from eating carbohydrates.

To begin burning fats for vitality, the general purpose of a keto diet — your body needs to consume any glucose that is available in your body initially.

There are a few sorts of discontinuous fasting conventions that will assist you with entering ketosis quicker.

In the event that you are an apprentice, skipping breakfast in the first part of the day is an extraordinary method to begin.

In the event that you are as of now keto-adjusted, fat fasting is a typical method to help with a weight loss level. This is the point at which you devour 80-90% of calories from fat for a set timeframe (close to three to five days) while restricting everything else. Doing so will permit your body to accelerate its digestion to consume increasingly fat.

#2: Decrease Stress

Ceaseless pressure will seriously block your body's capacity to enter ketosis. This is on the grounds that the pressure hormone cortisol hoists your glucose levels, which keeps your body from burning fats for vitality in light of the fact that there is a lot of sugar in the blood.

On the off chance that you are as of now experiencing a high-pressure period in your life, beginning the ketogenic diet may not be the best thought.

It's ideal to start this sustenance plan when you can downplay pressure, and you're ready to commit an enormous bit of your waking hours towards remaining in ketosis.

In the event that you certainly need to begin a keto diet currently, it's as yet possible. Simply make certain to find a way to reduce the worry in your life, for example, getting enough rest, practising normally, setting aside an effort to accomplish something you appreciate (like tuning in to your most loved digital broadcast) or embracing unwinding methods like profound breathing, contemplation or yoga.

#3: Prioritize Your Sleep

Poor rest will build levels of your pressure hormones. As clarified over, that you can forestall yourself from getting into fat-burning mode.

Women over 50 should have a go at Maintaining a legitimate rest plan on a keto diet where you hit the hay simultaneously regular will help improve your nature of rest.

It's basic to get at any rate seven to nine hours of rest each night. However, in case you're as of now getting route not as much as that, take a stab at downsizing by a half-hour consistently until you hit your rest objective.

Not getting enough rest can incredibly hurt your capacity to shed pounds.

Dozing in a moderately nippy room (around 65 degrees) alongside keeping a dull room will assist you with getting into a profound, remedial rest all the more habitually.

On the off chance that you experience difficulty resting, enhancing with a characteristic tranquillizer as melatonin can likewise do something amazing.

#4: Add More Salt To Your Diet

Numerous individuals have a negative shame with regards to how a lot of sodium you ought to be expanding every day. We have been encouraged that our sodium admission ought to be exceptionally low; however, this is regularly just the case on high starch counts calories.

This is on the grounds that higher carb eats less carbs normally implies more elevated levels of insulin. At the point when insulin levels are high, your kidneys start to hold sodium.

At the point when you embrace a low carb, high-fat eating regimen like the keto diet, insulin levels are a lot of lower and your body discharges progressively salt since there are no carbohydrates present in your body to spike insulin and clutch the sodium.

At the point when you're in ketosis, add an additional three to five grams (3,000 to 5,000 mg) of sodium in your eating routine.

This will assist you with avoiding electrolyte uneven characters. The healthiest approaches to get increasingly salt in your eating regimen include:

- Adding Himalayan ocean salt (or pink salt), which contains common follow minerals, to your water for the duration of the day

- Drinking natural bone stock ordinary

- •
- Sprinkling pink salt on every single one of your meals

- Eating low carb foods that normally contain sodium like cucumbers and celery.

- Eating salted macadamia nuts

#5: Exercise Frequently

Women over 50 should have a go at maintaining a normal exercise plan while on the keto diet can support your ketone levels and assist you with progressing into a low carb, high-fat way of life a lot speedier than without exercise. To get into ketosis, your body needs to dispose of any glucose present in the body.

Practicing utilizes various sorts of vitality for fuel including carbohydrates, fats and amino acids. The more regularly you exercise, the snappier your body exhausts its glycogen stores.

When your body has disposed of its glycogen stockpiles, it will search out different types of fuel and will go to fat for vitality through ketosis.

Make certain to fuse an exercise routine that incorporates both high force exercises related to low power consistent state exercises like strolling or running. This will assist you in adjusting your glucose and helps your body in entering ketosis.

Remember, this is a novice exercise for individuals who need to fuse a compelling exercise program to help with their excursion to ketosis.

#6: Stop Drinking Diet Soda and Using Sugar Substitutes

Because diet soft drink has zero calories doesn't mean it fits into your ketogenic diet plan.

Diet soft drinks utilize a few sugar substitutes that can move toward your body that a lot of sugar is entering the body. This can prompt expanded glucose levels.

Studies have indicated that the body may respond along these lines to some sugar substitutes as it would to customary sugar.

Also, when you load up on zero-calorie sugars, you're just going to build your longings for sweet foods and beverages later on. One of the enormous benefits of a keto diet is that you re-adjust your taste buds to long for healthy, low carb entire foods — however, this can't occur in case you're continually barraging them with sweet-tasting foods.

Rather than diet pop, shimmering water can be an extraordinary option without pointless sugar substitutes.

#7: Batch Cook

Clump preparing scrumptious keto meals will assist you with remaining on track with your keto macros consistently. In the event that you engineer your condition to support your objectives as opposed to attacking them, you're offering your resolve a reprieve, since it doesn't need to be solid notwithstanding allurement.

Clump concocting sets you for seven days of keto dishes, so you don't slip up when lunch or dinner opportunity arrives around.

#8: Drink Plenty of Water

Remaining hydrated is significant regardless of what diet you're on; however, you should give additional consideration when beginning on the ketogenic diet. This is on the grounds that your body discharges more water from your body when carbohydrates are absent.

Intend to drink half of your body weight in ounces of water at the base

Make certain to drink more on days where you are perspiring all the more frequently, for example, blistering summer days or after exceptional exercises.

#9: Consume Carbs From Vegetable Sources

It's critical to consolidate vegetables in your eating regimen to guarantee you're expending every essential supplement, including fibre, which is significant for keeping up a healthy gut (more on that later!).

You should focus on supplement thick, non-dull vegetables like:

- Kale
- Broccoli
- Cauliflower
- Spinach
- Cabbage
- Brussel grows

Non-bland vegetables are commonly low-calorie, as well. So in case you're the sort of individual who likes to feel genuinely full after a meal, it's critical to remember a lot of these vegetables for your eating regimen, so you're not eating a whole sack of macadamia nuts at a time.

While that would be tasty, it wouldn't be useful in case you're utilizing a keto diet to get more fit.

#10: Use MCT Oil Regularly

Enhancing with MCT (medium-chain triglyceride) oil will assist you with getting into ketosis regardless of whether your glycogen stockpiles aren't completely exhausted.

MCT's are promptly utilized into ketone bodies and utilized for vitality as opposed to experiencing your stomach for assimilation

While numerous individuals think coconut oil is equivalent to MCT, they are molecularly unique.

MCT oil is comprised of 100% medium-chain triglycerides — caprylic and capric acids — while coconut oil contains 35% long-chain triglycerides and 50% lauric corrosive. Coconut oil is just comprised of 15% medium-chain triglycerides. So your body needs to experience its stomach related tract to transform coconut oil into vitality while MCT oil is changed over legitimately into vitality.

#11: Improve Your Gut Micro biome

Gut health is connected to pretty much every framework in the body. A few researchs have demonstrated that your gut micro biome influences everything from your emotional well-being to your stomach related framework and a few different frameworks in the body.

At the point when you have healthy gut verdure, your body's hormones, metabolic adaptability, and insulin affectability become progressively productive. These procedures legitimately influence your body's capacity to change from carbohydrates to fats for vitality.

At the point when your metabolic adaptability is working ideally, your body can consistently adjust to low sugar, high-fat eating regimen. In any case, when your body is metabolically unbendable, it experiences issues using fats for vitality; rather, it will change over into body fat. Concentrating on improving your gut health will enormously affect the health of your body's metabolic adaptability.

Eating a low carb, high fat ketogenic diet additionally assists with your gut health. At the point when you wipe out carbs from your eating regimen, you're disposing of handled foods, which are known to hurt your gut microbiome.

Concentrating on improving your gut health can enormously improve your body's capacity to turn into an increasingly effective fat eliminator.

#12: Invest in a Food Scale

Gauging the food you eat can be an enormous distinction on the ketogenic diet, particularly as an amateur.

Numerous individuals like to eyeball the measure of food they're eating yet doing so can make you overeat and show you out of ketosis.

The distinction between burning glucose or ketones as your essential wellspring of fuel can be that one additional tablespoon of almond spread that you eyeballed.

For correlation, only two additional tablespoons of almond margarine turn out to an extra 200 calories and 6 grams of carbs.

When you become accustomed to what legitimate segments resemble, at that point, you can start to eyeball your meals.

#13: Use Exogenous Ketones

Like MCT oil, expending exogenous ketones resembles an alternate route to getting into ketosis.

The most well-known exogenous ketones available contain beta-hydroxybutyrate (BHB), which is the dynamic type of ketones that stream unreservedly in the blood and are effortlessly utilized by your body.

Taking a ketone supplement will radically help during the underlying periods of your ketogenic venture since you are flagging your body to begin utilizing ketones for vitality rather than carbohydrates.

You despite everything need to embrace a high fat, low carb diet to completely profit by along these lines of eating. However, exogenous ketones can kick you once again into ketosis significantly after an accidentally high starch meal.

It is likewise a compelling device for avoiding the keto influenza that is normal in learners.

While your body is as yet becoming acclimated to utilizing ketones, you can utilize an exogenous ketone to help dispense with the entirety of seasonal influenza-like side effects that come during the enlistment period of the ketogenic diet.

#14: Count Your Carbs

Estimating your starch admission is critical. Be cautious for shrouded carbohydrates in specific foods that may appear keto-accommodating, however, are really stacked with sugars.

Here are a few examples of keto foods that may have shrouded carbohydrates:

• Chicken wings stacked with grill or wild ox sauce

• Milk

• Most natural products (blueberries are fine in limited quantities)

-      Low-fat foods like yoghurt

-      Breaded meats

Make a point to take a gander at the nourishment realities of all that you eat until you comprehend where those concealed carbs are originating from.

You should just be devouring 50 grams most extreme in carbohydrates on the ketogenic diet.

While computing your carb check, you need to decide the net carbs of your all-out everyday admission.

All out carbs – Fiber = Net Carbs

The dependable general guideline is to devour 20 to 30 net carbs day by day. On the off chance that you exercise all the more oftentimes, you can pull off the upper limit and still remain in ketosis.

At the outset, it might appear as though the main thing you do is tally and track carbs throughout the day, yet we guarantee; it turns out to be progressively natural.

#15: Measure Your Ketones

Utilizing keto sticks or a glucose meter will give you criticism on whether you're following the eating routine accurately and in case you're quite a ketosis.

The most exact estimating apparatus is a glucose meter. It's additionally the most costly elective, which is the reason the vast majority are hindered from utilizing them day by day.

Keto sticks are additionally a decent option since they are modest. Remember, numerous individuals, guarantee that the keto sticks are not so much exact in light of the fact that the more you remain in ketosis, the more your body can use ketones for vitality as opposed to discharging it through your pee. So your ketone tally may show up low when it's really not.

#16: Always Have Convenient Snacks on Hand

Time is an immense factor with regards to adhering to the ketogenic diet. Numerous individuals are debilitated because of the measure of natively constructed meals you need to make.

An extraordinary solution for this is to plan the same number of keto-accommodating snacks as you can so you aren't going to helpful, carb substantial bites when you lack in time.

Here are a few examples of keto snacks you can take in a hurry:

- Hard bubbled eggs

- Beef jerky

- Premade guacamole

- Keto MCT Matcha Fat Bombs

- Pre-cooked bacon

#17: Clear Out Your Kitchen

The vast majority can adhere to a healthy keto diet in the event that they just approach healthy keto foods. Most individuals fall prey to starch loaded foods just on the grounds that they've neglected to expel them from their home.

Clearing out your kitchen and storeroom of all carbohydrates including bread, pasta, soft drinks, treats and rice will essentially drive you to adhere to your ketogenic diet.

It might sound radical from the outset, yet supplanting the entirety of your carbs, with the exception of no

#18: Be Prepared When Eating Out at Restaurants

At the point when you are first beginning the ketogenic diet, it very well may be troublesome distinctive what's keto-accommodating and so forth.

Yet, it gets simpler with time. Pretty much every café you go to will have a meal that is ketogenic diet benevolent, and with a little inventiveness, you will never need to depend on a carb substantial meal since you went out to eat with companions.

Here are the absolute most ideal approaches to remain keto when eating out:

- Breakfast — Always settle on eggs and bacon. Rather than going for hotcakes or toast, substitute it with more eggs and a green plate of mixed greens as an afterthought.

- Lunch — There are consistently serving of mixed greens options in practically any café you go to. Supplant the sugar-filled dressings with carefully olive oil and vinegar.

- Dinner — Every eatery will have a prevailing meat meal. In the event that you are going out for dinner, request their fattiest cut of steak, (for example, rib eye) and supplant the potatoes with an additional serving of vegetables.

It's additionally a good thought to take a gander at the menu already, so you recognize what the best options are.

Getting into the Keto Mindset that guarantees Keto Diet Success

I don't realize numerous weight control plans you've experienced, however, let me let you know, in the event that you don't have the correct attitude; odds are you're not going to succeed. Truth be told, in case you're similar to a great many people, your experience will fit a recognizable example. In the first place, you're completely amped up for the eating routine, and sufficiently sure, you follow the bearings intently.

On account of your cautious dietary rules above, and your energetic consistency, you begin losing a ton of pounds. Everything looks OK, isn't that so? This keeps up for perhaps a couple of more days or even a couple of more weeks. In any case, at some point or another, the pounds begin returning.

Next, things go from awful to more regrettable. You begin putting on more weight than when you started your eating regimen. Isn't the general purpose of starting to eat better to shed pounds? Unfortunately, most eating regimens are passages, in all honesty, to extra weight; talk about a disappointing circumstance.

The motivation behind why individuals experience this very well-known terrible example is on the grounds that they don't have the correct outlook. It doesn't make a difference whether you are attempting to receive the keto diet, the paleo diet, the Atkins diet, the Ornish, or some other loss program, without the correct outlook, you are playing the game to lose.

At any rate, you ought to receive three fundamental outlooks that will guarantee keto diet achievement.

Mentality #1

Expect that you can do it.

It's anything but difficult to get amped up for the tributes remembered for some eating routine books. You take a gander at the when pictures, and you and you get all siphoned up. If it's not too much trouble comprehend that a great deal of those photos is misrepresented. Truth be told, a lot of books that are extremely obscure even use photoshopped pictures.

I realize that it's difficult to accept that individuals would really do that, yet they do. So a smidgen of suspicion goes far. In any case, don't simply concentrate on the way that the eating regimen can work for others. Rather, understand the likelihood that the eating regimen can really work for you.

It's hard to believe, but it's true, you by and by, exclusively. In the event that you can't get that, and on the off chance that you can't acknowledge the probability of a specific weight-loss program sitting tight for you, at that point you're making things a lot harder on yourself. It resembles attempting to play b-ball and attempting to get the ball through the band.

In the event that in the rear of your head you're stating to yourself, "Others can shoot truly well, however not me," what might occur? You're shooting precision will go down. You're sabotaging yourself. You're making things pointlessly harder on yourself.

This is the reason it's essential to accept that you can make progress with the keto diet. Not the contextual investigation pictures, not the individuals are giving tributes, we are discussing you. In the event that you can't make this suspicion, at that point it will be an unpleasant street ahead for you.

Attitude #2

Start with what you have.

One basic motivation behind why individuals fall flat with counts calories is on the grounds that they imagine that they need to change into a totally extraordinary individual. On the other hand, they accept that their conditions or their circumstances need to change so significantly to guarantee achievement.

At the point when individuals think thusly, they're essentially simply giving themselves pardons for either not attempting, or for anticipating awful outcomes. Trust me. I can comprehend why individuals do this. On the off chance that you have been let somewhere near eating regimen after eating routine, it's anything but difficult to get tainted.

Truth be told, much of the time, it's extremely simple to anticipate disappointment. All things considered, you've experienced the natural procedure of at first shedding pounds, and afterwards getting everything back. It turns into an old story, and it won't be long before your heart gets broken once more.

This is the reason you feel that you should make a huge difference that you can change, to lay the basis for extreme achievement. Once more, you're making things superfluously harder on yourself. It doesn't need to be this way. You don't need to move paradise and earth to make ideal conditions.

You know why? Conditions are rarely great. There will never be the point at which your conditions will be perfect for you to guarantee achievement. You will need to face that challenge. You will need in any case what you have.

It doesn't make a difference what order level you have. It doesn't make a difference what else is going on in your life. It doesn't make a difference whether you like yourself. The only thing that is in any way important is that you are eager to get going in the first place what you have and accept that this will work for you.

Mentality #3

Make the most of your food as indicated by rules you pick

Another key "column" for keto diet achievement includes the issue of control. Many individuals come up short with eats fewer carbs on the grounds that they believe that they are putting a type of dietary straitjacket on themselves. For example, they don't regularly like a specific taste, yet since they're exchanging over to another eating routine, they compel themselves to like a specific scope of flavours.

You will scarcely believe, and it won't be long before your old self pops up. It won't be long before you return to how you typically eat. This is baffling. Maybe you are doing truly well, and you're making every one of these changes, and out of nowhere, your old self pulls you back. You end up where you started.

This is the reason it's extremely imperative to concentrate on making the most of your food. This isn't a trial. This isn't a type of discipline. This isn't a type of circumstance where you feel that you deny yourself. Rather, the keto diet ought to be a festival of taste. Everything comes down to making the most of your food as per keto rules.

You have first to pick the keto rules. You need to choose to go on the eating regimen initially, and afterwards you select depends on your current tastes. There's no compelling reason to become somebody else. There's no compelling reason to change your taste buds. There's no compelling reason to experience any of that. Rather, permit yourself to appreciate the flavour go that you are as of now encountering.

Presently listen to this, regardless of whether you have a sweet tooth, you will need to limit that. That is the main change, however, for everything else, regardless of whether you like acrid foods, salty foods, or unquestionably fatty foods, you ought to be fine. In any case, as long as you deal with your sweet tooth, you ought to be alright.

Keep the outlooks above on the off chance that you need to be effective with the keto diet. I'm not going to deceive you and state that you can embrace these mentalities overnight. All things considered, the manner in which you see things, and the manner in which you anticipate that things should play out have been with you for quite a while. You've become used to considering food a specific way.

Be that as it may, on the off chance that you change your outlook as per the three key columns above, embracing the keto diet will get simpler, and it is bound to adhere to a Healthy Keto Lifestyle.

Don't trust that things will quiet down.

Presently is the main time there is. There is no other time than the present moment, and there never will be.

Hanging tight for "things to quiet down" is only a type of hesitation.

There will never truly be a quiet, and regardless of whether there is, you would prefer not to squander it beginning another eating routine.

This last year, we have had some boisterous and sincerely attempting occasions – we lost some friends and family, my Mom got truly harmed, and nothing appeared to go easily.

Whatever your life seems as though right presently cut out the same number of carbs as you can.

And afterwards, do something very similar tomorrow and continue doing that. In the long run, you will be in Ketosis and make it into a propensity.

BENEFITS OF KETO FOR WOMEN ABOVE 50

Top Health Benefits of Keto for Women

The fundamental benefits of keto for women are support for weight loss and healthy hormone balance, the two of which are basic to life span and wellbeing.

Keto can assist women with getting in shape.

Ostensibly the most alluring advantage of keto for women is weight loss. Females will, in general, hold a decent measure of fat tissue around the waist and hips, which is frequently called "difficult" body fat.

While you can't really "focus on" a particular area of your body fat, keto can enable your body to turn out to be better at using fat for vitality and settle insulin levels, the two of which are gainful for fat loss.

By removing carbs, your body changes from burning sugar (glucose) for fuel to burning fat, from food and your body, for vitality. Additionally, the expansion in fat admission on the keto diet is commonly advantageous for females hoping to shed pounds since healthy fat sources, similar to nuts, coconut, and avocado will, in general, be exceptionally satisfying (which makes it simpler to eat less calories for the duration of the day).

Sugar, in actuality, isn't very filling and will in general urge individuals to overeat; clearly, that is not all that good for weight loss.

Continuously recollect, however, regardless of whether you follow the keto diet, you should be burning a larger number of calories than you expend so as to get more fit/body fat. This is a rule that applies to us all, paying little mind to your sexual orientation, and there's a lot of research supporting the significance of vitality balance for weight loss.

Keto can help treat indications of menopause.

Ongoing research recommends that as much as 50 million women in the United States are influenced by menopausal indications and that an expected 1.2 billion women worldwide will be in menopause or postmenopause constantly 2030. Side effects of menopause by and large include:

- Insomnia

- Hot flushes

- Night sweats

- Mood issue

- Unexpected weight gain

- Vaginal dryness

In present-day therapeutic settings, the side effects of menopause are normally treated through hormone treatment (by and large estrogen). Lamentably, hormone treatment can display symptoms/intricacies of its own and isn't appropriate for all women.

The keto diet may display a non-hormonal treatment for managing menopause by encouraging healthy hormonal parity (normally), accordingly balancing out vitality levels, encouraging healthy hunger, supporting moxie, and diminishing irritation all through the body.

At the point when you eat an eating regimen wealthy in healthy fats and low in sugar/dull carbs, you help reduce unpredictable swings in glucose and insulin, which thusly advances appropriate cortisol balance.

Cortisol awkwardness is one of the fundamental offenders of emotional episodes and weight gain.

Moreover, eating a high measure of healthy fats will enable your body to ingest and use nutrient D – a key forerunner to sex hormones. Be certain you expend ample measures of sinewy, micronutrient-rich veggies also since they give polyphenols and antioxidants which help reduce aggravation and advance alkalinity all through the body.

Keto can reduce food desires, disposition swings, and fatigue during your period.

Incomparable style to the keto diet managing manifestations of menopause, cutting carbs and eating progressively healthy fats can successfully constrict food desires, state of mind swings, and fatigue you may understanding during your period.

Since the premise of menopause and period is hormonal and biochemical changes, your eating regimen assumes a significant job in managing the side effects of them.

Keto for PMS

On the principal day of your cycle/period, both estrogen and progesterone are low. As you progress through the primary week, your ovaries begin to create more estrogen; this signals your body to back off and stop your period.

Presently your body advances into the follicular stage, as estrogen advises the ovaries to develop a follicle (which will end up being an egg). Estrogen levels keep on expanding for around two additional weeks so, all things considered, the ovulation happens.

When you enter the luteal stage (second 50% of your cycle), estrogen and progesterone arrive at their top following 10 days or somewhere in the vicinity. This is the point at which most females experience side effects of Premenstrual Syndrome (PMS). After the pinnacle, both estrogen and progesterone fall, setting off your period to start. This denotes the finish of one cycle and the start of the following one.

Side effects of PMS can be crippling to such an extent that females need to get a vacation from work or miss school. Normally, changing dietary propensities may help reduce these side effects by modifying lopsided concoction characteristics and supporting healthy estrogen and progesterone levels.

For instance, vacillations in serotonin levels are thought to assume a job in whimsical temperament states during PMS. Your body produces serotonin from the corrosive amino L-tryptophan, which is overwhelmingly found in turkey, red meat, eggs, fish, tofu, almonds, and different seeds. Adventitiously, those are on the whole foods that are keto-accommodating and incredible wellsprings of healthy fat also.

Moreover, since keto is commonly an extraordinary eating regimen for controlling hunger, it can help deal with those exceptional sugar/food desires you may be understanding from PMS. Enhancing with exogenous ketones is additionally a judicious choice on the off chance that you need something low in calories to help offer some relief from your craving.

Keto can help reduce swelling or inflammation

Females are particularly inclined to water maintenance and swelling during the luteal stage as estrogen and progesterone levels arrive at their pinnacle. It's essential to take note of that swelling, and other physical side effects, (for example, bosom delicacy) are totally normal during this time.

Numerous females feel like there is something "incorrectly" when they experience swelling and water maintenance during their cycle, yet actually, this is revealing to them their body is functioning as it should.

By and by, you can reduce the seriousness of swelling you experience by lessening sugar/carb admission, as glucose and glycogen are water-drawing in atoms. Fat, despite what might be expected, is hydrophobic, which means it repulses water.

In that capacity, the keto diet will, in general, reduce water maintenance and swelling.

Be cautious, however, as your body totally needs water and electrolytes for healthy capacity. It's not prescribed to utilize things like solution diuretics or limit your liquid admission since you're feeling enlarged.

Keto can assist you with deduction all the more plainly for the duration of the day.

Numerous individuals do the change to keto for mind boosting benefits of healthy fats and ketones. The keto diet can improve mental sharpness and lucidity for the duration of the day by encouraging healthy neuronal trustworthiness and expanding levels of cerebrum determined neurotrophic factor (BDNF).

Moreover, keto may help reduce incendiary procedures in the cerebrum and even lower the danger of subjective brokenness.

As opposed to eats less that are high in sugar (which can be neurotoxic), the keto diet seems to slow neurodegenerative procedures in the cerebrum.

As it were: ketones and certain healthy fats (like MCTs) are nootropics with neuroprotective properties. This is the reason numerous individuals decide to enhance with exogenous ketones as well as MCTs for the duration of the day when they feel that mid-evening droop going ahead.

SMALL ROUTINE OF EXERCISES FOR WOMEN OVER 50.

12 Best Workout Apps for Women Over 50

Women over 50 realize they have to improve their wellness levels; however can, in any case, make some hard memories fitting it into their bustling timetables. While they may hunger for the kinship that one encounters at an exercise centre or during a class, certain things could keep them away from engaging in them. Booking clashes are normal yet so is exploring the way of life of a specific exercise centre or class. Exercise applications can give the inspiration and assortment that women need to remain healthy while as yet meeting their different needs. We took a gander at what's available and recommended these as the absolute best exercise applications out there.

1. Yoga Poses

Yoga Poses offers you 250 yoga presents with going with video demos, changes for learners and clarifications about the benefits you can get involved in each posture. This free application is perfect in case you're progressively happy with practising or learning new stances in private.

A few women over age 50 have been rehearsing yoga for quite a long time, if not decades, while others come to it without precedent for their 50s.

One thing that is imperative to comprehend about yoga is that there is a wide range of kinds of styles. A few types of yoga may be too quick-paced, strenuous or truly trying for certain individuals, regardless of their age, while different styles are intended to be remedial and delicate. Except if you're an accomplished yogi, it's normally best to stay with the gentler types of yoga, which for the most part centre around extending and equalization more than on building quality and muscle.

2. Endomondo

The Endomondo application is free and basically transforms your iPhone into a fitness coach. Utilizing your telephone's GPS abilities, Endomondo screens your preferred movement — even fresh ones like kayaking, skiing and climbing — and conveys execution input. You can design courses in Google Maps, tune in to music and get consolation by means of texts from companions from inside the application.

3. Gixo

Gixo's slogan is Exercise Live and On Demand, which summarizes the application pleasantly. Regardless of whether you're voyaging or at home, you can join a live exercise bunch day and night. Look over classes that run 15, 30 or 40 minutes in length that are anything but difficult to fit into your bustling calendar. Tap into a library of pre-recorded classes all day, every day in any wellness level. With Gixo, it resembles having a fitness coach to work together with to assist you with arriving at your wellness objectives.

4. Day by day Burn

Unquestionably extraordinary compared to other exercise applications out there, and FREE, Daily Burn lets you flawlessly track both your caloric admission and your exercise yield in one intelligent spot. Remembered for the application is a calorie counter that lets you examine a food's standardized tag and get moment nourishing data. You can likewise stream in excess of 1,000 exercises running from learners to cutting edge.

5. Fitness Builder

Fitness Builder gives you the intensity of a fitness coach alongside the capacity to record and track your exercises so you can contrast your advancement and your companions. With FitnessBuilder Plus Access, you can look over in excess of 1,000 exercises and over 7,000 recordings and wellness pictures to guarantee your structure is right and the sky is the limit from there.

6. You Are Your Own Gym

Taking a shot at the reason that you don't have any equipment, You Are Your Own Gym is stuffed with 200 bodyweight exercises that tap into simply your own body's weight to be compelling. Accessible for Apple and Android gadgets, this application additionally incorporates how-to recordings and alterations so you can modify the exercises to your wellness level.

7. Yoga Wake Up

With the Yoga Wake Up application, you may be influenced to turn into a morning individual — regardless of whether you aren't at the present time. These simple routines are ones you can do directly from your bed and range from extends that jump-start the system, those that invigorate you, ones that expansion your careful breathing and that's only the tip of the iceberg.

8. SEVEN Minute Workout

The 7 Minute Workout application lets even the busiest women crush in exercise routines that are short, yet compelling. Utilizing a mix of cardio and quality preparing exercises that needn't bother with any exceptional equipment, the 7 Minute Workout likewise keeps tabs on your development to keep you both roused and tested.

9. Love seat to 5K Running App

On the off chance that running a 5K is on your pail list since you've outperformed the 50 years mark, it very well may be all around threatening to realize how to begin. That is the place the Couch to 5K Running App comes in. Straightforwardness into preparing with a nine-week program that makes them run three times each week for 30 minutes each time. Browse four virtual mentors with their own unmistakable characters to keep you spurred.

10. Pilates Anytime

Pilates Anytime takes the dubious jargon related to the training and separates each move plainly. You can observe every one the same number of times as you have to feel good without the weights that a gathering setting frequently brings. In case you're as of now a Pilates star, look over one of the 2,500 included classes that go from top picks like froth roller exercises, essential tangle routines, barre combination and that's only the tip of the iceberg.

11. My Fitness Pal

My Fitness Pal is your one-stop area for following your eating routine, exercise and caloric admission. On the off chance that you will likely get more fit — or shield weight from crawling up on you — notwithstanding getting fit, My Fitness Pal makes it quick and simple to check calories while giving a spot to log your exercise.

12. GymGoal

Adding weights to your exercises can assist you with holding bulk, adaptability and quality as you age. The beginning can be scary, yet the Gym Goal application is here to help. With your one-time acquisition of Gym Goal, you approach an amazing, customizable and expandable wellness application. Not exclusively will you get familiar with the correct structure for weight lifting, you'll additionally approach a developing library of exercises that can be changed dependent on both your capacities and your objectives.

Transforming your cell phone into a wellness instrument is made simpler with the plenty of applications accessible today. The best exercise applications are the ones you'll really utilize. The above determinations are intended to give you a sample of the different alternatives you can take advantage of to meet your health objectives.

• Strength preparing. Great weight preparing routines for women over 50 incorporate lifting weights, just as exercises that include the utilization of obstruction, for example, Pilates or working out with opposition groups.

Squats with Chair

Another weight-bearing exercise that is anything but difficult to do at home is squats with a seat. During this exercise, you squat over a seat as though you were going to plunk down, however, don't reach the seat. Rather, you remain back up and rehash the procedure on numerous occasions.

Squats help tone your lower body, yet they can likewise help improve balance. At the point when you begin, you may think that it's most straightforward to play out the exercise with your hands and arms reached out before you.

Chest Fly

Women will, in general, have extremely feeble and immature chest muscles. The chest fly is a weightlifting exercise that fortifies those muscles.

To do the exercise, you'll need a couple of hand weights. Lie on the floor, or a tangle, level on your back, with your knees bowed and your feet level on the ground. Take one weight in each hand and raise your arms over your chest.

Gradually, open your arms out to the side, bringing down your arms and wrists toward the floor — yet don't really contact the ground. Keep a slight twist in your elbows, so you don't bolt out your arms. Raise your arms back up and rehash.

•

Aerobic/cardiovascular. Vigorous or cardiovascular exercises are now and then called perseverance exercises since you should keep up them for in any event 10 minutes. During oxygen consuming exercise, your pulse and breathing should increment. However you should, in any case, have the option to carry on a discussion with an exercise mate. Strolling, running and swimming are, for the most part, examples of oxygen-consuming exercise.

•   Stretching. Extending exercises help improve or look after adaptability, diminishing the danger of damage to the muscles or joints. Yoga is a well-known kind of extending exercise.

•   Balance. As you get more seasoned, the danger of falling increments. Exercises that help improve or keep up equalization can reduce your danger of falls. An equalization exercise can be as basic as remaining on one foot.

In spite of the fact that there are four separate classes of exercise, it's critical to comprehend exercise doesn't occur in a vacuum. For instance, when you play out an oxygen-consuming exercise, for example, strolling, you aren't simply reinforcing your cardiovascular framework, yet additionally fabricating your leg muscles. A few kinds of solidarity preparing exercises can likewise help stretch the muscles or improve your equalization.

13. SWIMMING

Swimming is one case of a magnificent exercise for women over 50. While a lot of different exercises, for example, running and strolling, can put a great deal of strain on your joints, swimming is low-sway. The water goes about as a pad and backing around you, keeping pressure off of your joints.

Try not to be tricked by its tenderness, however. Swimming will give you a complete body exercise. It will assist you with building perseverance while it reinforces the muscles on your upper and lower body and in your centre. Moreover, by building up your centre, swimming can likewise help improve your equalization, lessening the danger of falls when you're back ashore.

MEAL PLAN FOR 14DAYS WITH RECIPES FOR BREAKFAST, LUNCH DINNER AND SNACKS

14-Day Clean-Eating Meal Plan: 1,200 Calories

This simple clean-eating meal plan for weight loss highlights healthy entire foods and points of confinement prepared things to assist you with refocusing with healthy propensities.

In the event that you have an inclination that your healthy propensities have gotten off track, this basic interpretation of a spotless eating meal plan can assist you with returning to the dietary patterns that assist you with feeling your best. Over the course of this 14-day diet plan, you'll get your fill of entire healthy foods-some that you'll prepare without any preparation and others that you can purchase from the store

7 Tips for Clean Eating

The meals and snacks right now make them feel stimulated, fulfilled, and great about what's on your plate. Furthermore, at 1,200 calories, this eating regimen meal plan will set you up to lose as much as 4 pounds over the 2 weeks.

Clean-Eating Meal Plan for Beginners

In case you're new to clean eating, the reason is straightforward—and following a meal plan (or basically utilizing it for motivation) can make it considerably more obvious what it's everything about. Clean-gobbling is an extraordinary method to up your admission of bravo foods (like entire grains, lean protein, healthy fats and a lot of leafy foods) while restricting the stuff that can cause you to feel not very good in enormous sums (think refined carbs, liquor, included sugars and hydrogenated fats).

Here at EatingWell, we approach clean-eating reasonably. While all foods can be a piece of a healthy eating regimen, now and then you simply need to hit reset and spotlight on eating a greater amount of the healthy foods you might be holding back on. With 14 days of healthy meals and bites, this simple-to-follow clean-eating meal plan is an extraordinary way to get a greater amount of those bravo foods.

Where you can plan to eat huge amounts of flavorful clean-eating foods, similar to what you'll discover right now.

Week 1

The most effective method to Meal Prep Your Week of Meals:

A little prep toward the start of the week goes far to make your week ahead simple.

1.   Make a twofold clump of the Lemon-Tahini Dressing. You'll utilize it during the time for lunch and dinner. Store right now serving of mixed greens dressing holder.

Cook a twofold clump of the Easy Brown Rice to use consistently. Store in an enormous glass meal-prep holder. Since Day 1's dinner—the Kale Salad with Beets and Wild Rice—calls for wild rice, you can decide to either prepare a greater cluster of wild rice or swap in dark coloured rice in the formula, so you're not making two unique grains of rice.

Day 1

Breakfast (287 calories)

• 1 serving Muesli with Raspberries

Clean-Eating Shopping Tip: When purchasing muesli, search for a brand that doesn't have included sugars, which detract from the healthy integrity of this entire grain breakfast.

A.M. Bite (62 calories)

• 1 medium orange

Lunch (360 calories)

- 4 cups White Bean and Veggie Salad

- P.M. Bite (95 calories)

- 1 medium apple

Dinner (420 calories)

- 4 cups (1/2 servings) Kale Salad with Beets and Wild Rice

- 1 serving Balsamic-Dijon Chicken

Meal-Prep Tip: Save 1 serving Balsamic-Dijon Chicken (1/2 bosom) for lunch of Day 2.

Day by day Totals: 1,224 calories, 61 g protein, 153 g carbohydrates, 40 g fibre, 47 g fat, 1,400 mg sodium.

Day 2

Breakfast (270 calories)

• 1 serving Avocado-Egg Toast

Clean-Eating Shopping Tip: Use grew grain bread as your bread for these next about fourteen days as it's made without included sugars, dissimilar to many locally acquired bread. Additionally, on the off chance that you intend to top your egg toast with hot sauce, search for a brand that is made without included sugars.

A.M. Bite (101 calories)

• 1 medium pear

Lunch (353 calories)

- 2 cups blended greens

- 1/2 cup hacked cucumber

- 1/2 Balsamic-Dijon Chicken bosom, hacked

- 2 Tbsp. Lemon-Tahini Dressing

- 2 Tbsp. sunflower seeds

- Consolidate greens, cucumber and chicken and top with dressing and sunflower seeds.

- P.M. Bite (62 calories)

- 1 medium orange

Dinner (439 calories)

- 1 serving cup Squash and Red Lentil Curry

- 1/2 cup Easy Brown Rice

Meal-Prep Tip: Save a 1 cup serving of rice to have for dinner on Day 3.

Every day Totals: 1,225 calories, 63 g protein, 147 g carbohydrates, 33 g fibre, 46 g fat, 1,965 mg sodium.

Day 3

Breakfast (287 calories)

• 1 serving Muesli with Raspberries

A.M. Bite (62 calories)

• 1 medium orange

Lunch (326 calories)

• 1 serving cups Squash and Red Lentil Curry

P.M. Bite (92 calories)

• 12 almonds

Dinner (439 calories)

• 1 serving Asian Tilapia with Stir-Fried Green Beans

• 1 cup Easy Brown Rice

Every day Totals: 1,206 calories, 62 g protein, 174 g carbohydrates, 37 g fibre, 48 g fat, 1,444 mg sodium.

Day 4

Breakfast (257 calories)

- 1/2 cup moved oats, cooked in 1 cup milk

- 1 medium plum, hacked

- Cook oats and top with plum and a touch of cinnamon.

- A.M. Bite (95 calories)

- 1 medium apple

Lunch (325 calories)

• 1 serving Veggie and Hummus Sandwich

Clean-Eating Shopping Tip: Double-check the fixing list on hummus to ensure you're picking one without included sugars or overabundance sodium. You can likewise take a stab at making your own. EatingWell's Garlic Hummus is both simple and delectable.

P.M. Tidbit (105 calories)

• 1 medium banana

Dinner (432 calories)

• 1 serving Sheet-Pan Chicken and Brussels Sprouts

• 1/2 cups blended greens dressed with 2 Tbsp. Lemon-Tahini Dressing

Every day Totals: 1,214 calories, 58 g protein, 166 g carbohydrates, 32 g fibre, 41 g fat, 1,553 mg sodium.

Day 5

Breakfast (290 calories)

• 1 serving Peanut Butter-Banana Cinnamon Toast

Clean-Eating Shopping Tip: When picking a locally acquired nutty spread, avoid brands with included sugars and trans fats.

A.M. Tidbit (32 calories)

• 1/2 cup raspberries

Lunch (360 calories)

• 4 cups White Bean and Veggie Salad

Dinner (543 calories)

• 1 serving Pork Chops with Garlicky Broccoli

Day by day Totals: 1,225 calories, 54 g protein, 102 g carbohydrates, 30 g fibre, 71 g fat, 1,175 mg sodium.

Day 6

Breakfast (257 calories)

- 1/2 cup moved oats, cooked in 1 cup milk

- 1 medium plum, cleaved

- Cook oats and top with plum and a spot of cinnamon.

- A.M. Tidbit (101 calories)

- 1 medium pear

Lunch (325 calories)

• 1 serving Veggie and Hummus Sandwich

- P.M. Tidbit (62 calories)

- 1 medium orange

- Dinner (543 calories)

- 1 serving Cauliflower rice-stuffed Peppers

- 2 cups blended greens dressed with 1 Tbsp. Citrus Vinaigrette

Meal-Prep Tip: You'll utilize the rest of the Citrus Vinaigrette one week from now.

Every day Totals: 1,203 calories, 57g protein, 146 g carbohydrates, 31 g fibre, 49 g fat, 1,120 mg sodium.

Day 7

Breakfast (307 calories)

• 2 cups Jason Mraz's Avocado Green Smoothie

A.M. Bite (35 calories)

• 1 clementine

Lunch (352 calories)

• 2 1/4 cup Tomato, Cucumber and White-Bean Salad with Basil Vinaigrette

• 1 cut grew grain bread, toasted and bested with 1 Tbsp. hummus

Meal-Prep Tip: Save a serving of the Tomato, Cucumber and White-Bean Salad with Basil Vinaigrette to have for lunch on Day 10. Store the dressing independently.

P.M. Bite (30 calories)

• 1 plum

Dinner (490 calories)

• 1/2 cups Mexican Cabbage Soup

• 2 cups No-Cook Black Bean Salad

Meal-Prep Tip: Save a 1-cup serving of the No-Cook Black Bean Salad to have for lunch on Day 9. Store the dressing independently and hold on to add until prepared to eat. Get together 2 servings of the Mexican Cabbage Soup in a watertight holder.

Every day Totals: 1,214 calories, 35 g protein, 163 g carbohydrates, 48 g fibre, 55 g fat, 1,365 mg sodium.

Week 2

The most effective method to Meal Prep Your Week of Meals:

A little prep toward the start of the week goes far to make your week ahead simple.

1.   Make a clump of the Meal-Prep Sheet-Pan Chicken Thighs and Basic Quinoa while setting up the Greek Kale Salad with Quinoa and Chicken formula for dinner on Day 8. Along these lines, you'll have leftover chicken and quinoa to use during the week. Store leftovers of the chicken and quinoa independently in enormous glass meal-prep compartments.

Day 8

Breakfast (338 calories)

• 1 serving Scrambled Eggs with Vegetables

A.M. Bite (119 calories)

• 1/4 cup hummus

• 1 cup cut cucumber

Lunch (325 calories)

• 1 serving Veggie and Hummus Sandwich

P.M. Bite (30 calories)

• 1 plum

Dinner (302 calories)

• 1 serving Greek Kale Salad with Quinoa and Chicken

Night Snack (102 calories)

• 1 serving Broiled Mango

Every day Totals: 1,216 calories, 58 g protein, 121 g carbohydrates, 26 g fibre, 60 g fat, 1,816 mg sodium.

Day 9

Breakfast (307 calories)

• 2 cups Jason Mraz's Avocado Green Smoothie

A.M. Bite (35 calories)

• 1 clementine

Lunch (328 calories)

- 1/2 cups Mexican Cabbage Soup

- 1 cup No-Cook Black Bean Salad

P.M. Bite (92 calories)

- 3/4 cup Kiwi and Mango with Fresh Lime Zest

Dinner (453 calories)

- 1 cup riced cauliflower, warmed

- 1 serving Soy-Lime Roasted Tofu

- 2 cups Colorful Roasted Sheet-Pan Veggies

- 1 Tbsp. Citrus Vinaigrette

Top riced cauliflower with tofu, veggies and shower with the vinaigrette.

Day by day Totals: 1,216 calories, 44 g protein, 149 g carbohydrates, 42 g fibre, 59 g fat, 1,248 mg sodium.

Day 10

Breakfast (290 calories)

- 1 serving Peanut Butter-Banana Cinnamon Toast

A.M. Tidbit (64 calories)

• 1 cup raspberries

Lunch (370 calories)

• 1 serving Chicken and Apple Kale Wraps

P.M. Tidbit (92 calories)

• 1 plum

• 8 almonds

Dinner (402 calories)

• 1 serving Panko-Crusted Pork Chops with Asian Slaw

Day by day Totals: 1,217 calories, 72 g protein, 127 g carbohydrates, 29 g fibre, 50 g fat, 1,133 mg sodium.

Day 11

Breakfast (270 calories)

• 1 serving Avocado-Egg Toast

A.M. Tidbit (64 calories)

• 1 cup raspberries

Lunch (302 calories)

• 1 serving Greek Kale Salad with Quinoa and Chicken

P.M. Tidbit (95 calories)

• 1 medium apple

Dinner (478 calories)

• 1 serving Salmon and Asparagus with Lemon-Garlic Butter Sauce

• 1 cup Basic Quinoa

Meal-Prep Tip: Cook a hard-bubbled egg today around evening time, so it's prepared for your P.M. Nibble on Day 12.

Day by day Totals: 1,209 calories, 68 g protein, 128 g carbohydrates, 28 g fibre, 50 g fat, 1,233 mg sodium.

Day 12

Breakfast (290 calories)

• 1 serving Peanut Butter-Banana Cinnamon Toast

A.M. Bite (96 calories)

• 1 clementine

• 8 almonds

Lunch (344 calories)

   •   1/2 cups Mexican Cabbage Soup

   •   2 cups blended greens

   •   1 Tbsp. Citrus Vinaigrette

   •   2 Tbsp. sunflower seeds

   •   Hurl greens in vinaigrette. Top with sunflower seeds.

P.M. Bite (78 calories)

• 1 hard-bubbled egg, prepared with a squeeze every one of salt and pepper

Dinner (408 calories)

• 1 serving Spaghetti Squash and Meatballs

Day by day Totals: 1,216 calories, 60 g protein, 124 g carbohydrates, 30 g fibre, 56 g fat, 1,463 mg sodium.

Day 13

Breakfast (264 calories)

- 1 cup nonfat plain Greek yoghurt

- 1/4 cup muesli

- 1/4 cup blueberries

- A.M. Tidbit (70 calories)

- 2 clementines

Lunch (325 calories)

- 1 serving Veggie and Hummus Sandwich

- P.M. Tidbit (95 calories)

- 1 medium apple

Dinner (446 calories)

- 1 serving Zucchini Noodles with Avocado Pesto and Shrimp

Day by day Totals: 1,200 calories, 68 g protein, 133 g carbohydrates, 31 g fibre, 52 g fat, 1,102 mg sodium.

Day 14

Breakfast (270 calories)

- 1 serving Avocado-Egg Toast

- A.M. Tidbit (70 calories)

- 2 clementines

Lunch (378 calories)

- 2 1/4 cup Tomato, Cucumber and White-Bean Salad with Basil Vinaigrette

- 1 cut grew grain bread, toasted and beat with 2 Tbsp. hummus

- P.M. Tidbit (30 calories)

- 1 plum

Dinner (458 calories)

- 1 serving Fish with Coconut-Shallot Sauce

- 1/2 cup Basic Quinoa

- 2 cups blended greens beat with 1 Tbsp. Citrus Vinaigrette

Every day Totals: 1,207 calories, 61 g protein, 113 g carbohydrates, 27 g fibre, 60 g fat, 1,146 mg sodium.

Clean-Eating Meal Plan for winter

Right now eating meal plan for winter, You will comprehend what to eat to get more fit, with seven days of delightful and supplement pressed entire foods.

Right now eating meal plan for winter, you'll discover an abundance of regular winter produce that will assist you with eating healthy during the cold winter months.

7 Tips for Clean Eating

Here at EatingWell, we take a reasonable and proof-based way to deal with clean eating. Just eat a greater amount of the food that does your body great and less of the food that can be hurtful to your health. This arrangement tells you the best way to eat progressively supplement thick foods (like entire grains, natural products, vegetables, lean protein, lentils, beans and healthy fats like nuts and seeds) and less of the supplement lacking food (like handled foods and those with overabundance included sugar and hydrogenated fats just as liquor and refined carbohydrates). Your 7-day clean-eating meal plan will warm you from the back to front as you appreciate fibre-rich and antioxidant-rich simple clean-eating recipes to keep you full and fulfilled and your safe framework murmuring all through the winter months.

Every day of this spotless eating meal plan for winter times in at 1,200 calories, yet changes have been incorporated for 1,500-calorie days and 2,000-calorie days, contingent upon your necessities. Searching for a spotless eating meal plan for an alternate season?

Clean-Eating Food List for Winter

These are the foods to eat a greater amount of this winter, which we made certain to remember for this healthy meal plan.

- Brown rice

- Brussels grows

- Kale

- Tahini

- Chickpeas

- Garlic

- Cauliflower

- Butter beans

- Red potatoes

- Red onion

- Spinach

- Great northern beans

- Carrots

- Ginger

- Butternut squash

- Lentils

- Whole-wheat pasta

- Pomegranate

- Walnuts

- Pears

- Clementines

- Salmon

- Chicken

- Warming flavours, like smoked paprika, curry powder and cumin

Cleaning-Eating Foods List

7-Day Clean-Eating Meal Plan for Winter: 1,200 Calories

An entire seven day stretch of simple-to-make meals, in addition, to prepare ahead notes for making the bustling weekdays less upsetting.

The most effective method to Meal-Prep Your Week of Meals:

- Make the Mango-Date Energy Bites have for snacks consistently. Store in the cooler for 3 days or freeze for as long as 3 months.

- Prepare the Brussels Sprouts Salad with Crunchy Chickpeas to have for lunch on Days 2 through 5.

- Prepare the Muffin-Tin Quiches with Smoked Cheddar and Potato to have for breakfast on Days 2, 4 and 6. Independently enclose by plastic and refrigerate for as long as 3 days or freeze for as long as a multi-month. To warm, expel plastic, enclose by a paper towel and microwave on High for 30 to 60 seconds.

Day 1

Breakfast (262 calories)

- 1 serving Peanut Butter and Chia Berry Jam English Muffin

- A.M. Tidbit (95 calories)

- 1 medium apple

Lunch (325 calories)

- 1 serving Veggie and Hummus Sandwich

- P.M. Tidbit (73 calories)

- 1 Mango-Date Energy Bite

Dinner (427 calories)

- 1 serving Grilled Cauliflower Steaks with Almond Pesto and Butter Beans

Day by day Totals: 1,182 calories, 38 g protein, 152 g carbs, 37 g fibre, 54 g fat, 1,394 mg sodium

To make it 1,500 calories: Add 1 medium pear to breakfast, add 8 pecan parts to A.M. tidbit, and increment P.M. nibble to 2 Mango-Date Energy Bites.

To make it 2,000 calories: Add 1 medium pear and 1 tablespoon nutty spread to breakfast, add 16 pecan parts to A.M. nibble, increment P.M. nibble to 2 Mango-Date Energy Bites, include 1 entire wheat dinner move to dinner and include 1 cup low-fat plain Greek yoghurt and 1 clementine as a night nibble.

Day 2

Breakfast (272 calories)

- 1 serving Muffin-Tin Quiches with Smoked Cheddar and Potato

- 1 clementine

- A.M. Bite (73 calories)

- 1 Mango-Date Energy Bite

Lunch (337 calories)

- 1 serving Brussels Sprouts Salad with Crunchy Chickpeas

- P.M. Bite (166 calories)

- 1 cup low-fat plain Greek yoghurt

Dinner (344 calories)

- 1 serving Tuscan White Bean Soup

- 1 entire wheat dinner roll

Day by day Totals: 1,192 calories, 67 g protein, 129 g carbs, 40 g fibre, 48 g fat, 1,496 mg sodium

To make it 1,500 calories: Increase breakfast to 2 servings Muffin-Tin Quiches with Smoked Cheddar and Potato and add 1 clementine to P.M. nibble.

To make it 2,000 calories: Increase breakfast to 2 servings Muffin-Tin Quiches with Smoked Cheddar and Potato, include 1 clementine and 6 pecan parts to P.M. tidbit, and increment dinner to 2 servings Tuscan White Bean Soup.

Day 3

Breakfast (262 calories)

- 1 serving Peanut Butter and Chia Berry Jam English Muffin

- A.M. Tidbit (101 calories)

- 1 medium pear

Lunch (337 calories)

- 1 serving Brussels Sprouts Salad with Crunchy Chickpeas

- P.M. Tidbit (73 calories)

- 1 Mango-Date Energy Bite

Dinner (439 calories)

- 1 serving Squash and Red Lentil Curry
- 1 serving Easy Brown Rice

Day by day Totals: 1,212 calories, 39 g protein, 179 g carbs, 43 g fibre, 46 g fat, 1, 428 mg sodium

To make it 1,500 calories: Add 1 cup plain low-fat Greek yoghurt to A.M. nibble, increment P.M. nibble to 2 Mango-Date Energy Bites, and include 2 clementines as a night nibble.

To make it 2,000 calories: Add 1 cup plain low-fat Greek yoghurt to A.M. nibble, increment P.M. nibble to 2 Mango-Date Energy Bites, add 1 medium apple to P.M. nibble, increment dinner to 2 servings Squash and Red Lentil Curry, and include 3 clementines as a night nibble.

Day 4

Breakfast (272 calories)

- 1 serving Muffin-Tin Quiches with Smoked Cheddar and Potato

- 1 clementine

- A.M. Tidbit (95 calories)

- 1 medium apple

Lunch (337 calories)

- 1 serving Brussels Sprouts Salad with Crunchy Chickpeas

- P.M. Tidbit (147 calories)

- 2 Mango-Date Energy Bites

Dinner (371 calories)

- 1 serving Roasted Butternut Squash Salad with Burrata

- 1 entire wheat dinner roll

Day by day Totals: 1,222 calories, 40 g protein, 134 g carbs, 27 g fibre, 67 g fat, 1,471 mg sodium

Meal-Prep Tip: Prepare Slow-Cooker Mediterranean Chicken and Orzo at night on Day 4 and refrigerate to appreciate for dinner on Day 5 and for lunch on Day 6.

To make it 1,500 calories: Increase breakfast to 2 servings Muffin-Tin Quiches with Smoked Cheddar and Potato and add 1 clementine to P.M. nibble.

To make it 2,000 calories: Increase breakfast to 2 servings Muffin-Tin Quiches with Smoked Cheddar and Potato, include 1 cup plain low-fat Greek yoghurt to A.M. nibble, add 3 clementines to P.M. bite, and increment dinner to incorporate 2 entire wheat dinner rolls.

Day 5

Breakfast (262 calories)

- 1 serving Peanut Butter and Chia Berry Jam English Muffin

- A.M. Bite (101 calories)

- 1 medium pear

Lunch (337 calories)

- 1 serving Brussels Sprouts Salad with Crunchy Chickpeas

- P.M. Bite (166 calories)

- 1 cup low-fat plain Greek yoghurt

Dinner (353 calories)

- 1 serving Slow-Cooker Mediterranean Chicken and Orzo

- 1 entire wheat dinner roll

Day by day Totals: 1,218 calories, 76 g protein, 151 g carbs, 37 g fibre, 40 g fat, 1,311 mg sodium

Meal-Prep Tip: Refrigerate 1 serving of the Slow-Cooker Mediterranean Chicken and Orzo to have for lunch on Day 6.

To make it 1,500 calories: Add 1 tablespoon nutty spread to breakfast, add 1 medium apple to lunch and include 8 pecan parts and 1 medium apple to P.M. nibble.

To make it 2,000 calories: Add 1 tablespoon nutty spread to breakfast, TK lunch add 2 clementines to lunch, include 16 pecan parts and 1 medium apple to P.M. tidbit and increment dinner to 2 servings Slow-Cooker Mediterranean Chicken and Orzo

Day 6

Breakfast (273 calories)

- 1 serving Muffin-Tin Quiches with Smoked Cheddar and Potato

- 1 clementine

- A.M. Bite (147 calories)

- 2 Mango-Date Energy Bites

Lunch (278 calories)

- 1 serving Slow-Cooker Mediterranean Chicken and Orzo

- P.M. Bite (64 calories)

- 1 cup raspberries

Dinner (447 calories)

- 1 serving Roasted Salmon with Smoky Chickpeas and Greens

Day by day Totals: 1,208 calories, 84 g protein, 109 g carbs, 25 g fibre, 50 g fat, 1,557 mg sodium

To make it 1,500 calories: Increase A.M. nibble to 2 servings Mango-Date Energy Bites, increment lunch to 2 servings Slow-Cooker Mediterranean Chicken and Orzo and include 1 cup plain low-fat Greek yoghurt and 2 clementines to P.M. nibble.

To make it 2,000 calories: Increase breakfast to 2 servings Muffin-Tin Quiches with Smoked Cheddar and Potato, increment A.M. nibble to 3 servings Mango-Date Energy Bites, includes 1 entire wheat dinner roll and 1 little apple to lunch, and include 16 pecan parts, 1 cup plain low-fat Greek yoghurt and 2 clementines to P.M. nibble.

Day 7

Meal-Prep Tip: Prepare the Slow-Cooker Curried Butternut Squash Soup toward the beginning of the day of Day 7 to have for dinner.

Breakfast (262 calories)

- 1 serving Peanut Butter and Chia Berry Jam English Muffin

- A.M. Tidbit (70 calories)

- 2 clementines

Lunch (325 calories)

- 1 serving Veggie and Hummus Sandwich

- P.M. Tidbit (147 calories)

- 2 Mango-Date Energy Bites

Dinner (380 calories)

- 2 servings Slow-Cooker Curried Butternut Squash Soup

- 1 entire wheat dinner roll

Day by day Totals: 1,183 calories, 33 g protein, 163 g carbs, 33 g fibre, 54 g fat, 1,760 mg sodium

To make it 1,500 calories: Add 1 tablespoon nutty spread and 1 little apple to breakfast, increment A.M. nibble to 2 clementines in addition to 8 pecan parts, and add 1 teaspoon spread to the entire wheat dinner move at dinner.

To make it 2,000 calories: Increase breakfast to 2 servings Peanut Butter and Chia Berry Jam English Muffin and add 1 medium apple to breakfast, increment A.M. nibble to 2 clementines in addition to 10 pecan parts, and include 1 cup plain low-fat Greek yoghurt and 8 pecan parts to P.M. nibble.

BEST Meal Prep Recipes for breakfast, lunch or dinner with a couple of treat recipes snuck in there!

BEST Meal Prep Recipes for breakfast, lunch or dinner with a couple of pastry recipes snuck in there! Simple healthy recipes to get ready for the week that is ensured to keep you on track.

Folks, the recent weeks have been a compressed lesson again at having an infant. I got past the primary kid, and recall the initial a half year being fierce. However, at that point after those a half year, you at long last feel like your head is leaving the water, and you're back to yourself once more. All things considered, I'm unquestionably experiencing that at the present time.

Which implies each opportunity I find a workable pace I attempt to exploit. Things like tidying up around the house, or making a cluster of brownies with my child, doing schoolwork, playing a round of SORRY or making a meal. Or on the other hand, TAKING A SHOWER AND BLOW DRYING MY HAIR. Things that appear to be difficult to save time for; however, once I do them, I feel like myself once more.

These Meal Prep Recipes are an extraordinary method to assist you with planning for the week, to keep things healthy and leave you with delightful meals to eat up. However, above all else they are going to assist you with resting easy thinking about yourself, the things you are placing in your body and that you're remaining on track. Bon Appetit companions! I trust you appreciate!

BREAKFAST

Straightforward No Bake Chocolate Peanut Butter Energy Balls pressed with protein to keep you full more and pose a flavour like a Peanut Butter Cookie! Indeed, please!

New Almond Oat Raspberry Bars with a scrumptious disintegrate beating! These Raspberry Bars are sweet, tart, thoroughly fulfilling and righteous at 129 calories a bar! {gluten free, dairy-free, and vegan}

These Instant Pot hard bubbled eggs turn out astonishing inevitably!

4 Easy Smoothie Packs Recipes that can be made ahead and solidified for speedy use! Every smoothie is stacked with supplements, protein and fibre. Additionally, are kid endorsed.

These simple Snickerdoodle Energy Balls are made in a blender and afterwards abounded in a cinnamon coconut sugar outside. They taste simply like snickerdoodle treats and are the ideal breakfast, post-exercise nibble or late-night treat.

DINNER

Gluten-Free Roasted Veggie Balsamic Chicken Grain Bowls – a simple meal prep formula or weeknight dinner for the week. Heaps of veggies, light, delightful, simple to make with 28 grams of protein and under 350 calories a serving!

Have you been wanting to figure out how to meal prep your lunches, however, are a piece overwhelmed at making sense of what fixings go together? This Mix and Match Meal Prepping is a simple equation for eating made rapidly and flavorful.

1 Hour Roasted Chicken slathered in a garlic herb spread that will make you swoon. This simple cooked chicken formula is destined to be another family top pick, prep toward the end of the week and appreciate throughout the entire week!

Healthy Chicken Shawarma Quinoa Bowls with an excessively simple hack for making make-ahead lunches for work or school. The flavours are crazy!!

Discard the exhausting sandwiches and make yourself something genuinely heavenly for lunch with these Chickpea Gyro Lunch Boxes! In less than 30 minutes, you'll eat prepared for the week.

Cooked garlic and kale spaghetti squash with sun-dried tomatoes and pecans make for a soothing, low-carb meal requiring just 5 primary fixings! Besides the formula is easy to plan!

Taco Cones are the ideal method to change your family-most loved taco night into a snappy, compact, get an and-go meal! Our DIY Ta-Cones can even be prepared ahead – a simple make-ahead dinner formula that you can rewarm throughout the entire week, at whatever point your family is prepared to eat.

This healthy, gluten-free chicken burrito bowl formula can be made early, so it's all set for occupied days. It's a without dairy scrumptious work area lunch alternative!

Simple SWEET POTATO BLACK BEAN QUINOA BOWLS

bested with a lively Cilantro Dressing you'll need to pour everywhere. Make all the veggies early and prep these dishes to appreciate consistently!

Simple Thai Chicken Grain Bowl showered with a Creamy Peanut Dressing. These Grain Bowls are loaded up with veggies, thai flavours, 17 grams of protein and meet up in a short time.

These bricklayer container zucchini lasagnas are the ideal, compact, healthy meal! They're low carb, gluten-free, pressed with protein and immaculate to prepare ahead to get and go!

Cooked Vegetable Grain Bowls – a gluten-free grain bowl loaded up with spiced broiled vegetables at that point covered in a smooth Tzatziki Sauce. A meal your family will love and ideal for meatless Monday!

9 781667 153513